SECOND EDITION

STATISTICS FOR NURSING

A PRACTICAL APPROACH

Elizabeth Heavey, PhD, RN, CNM
Associate Professor of Nursing
SUNY College at Brockport
Brockport, New York

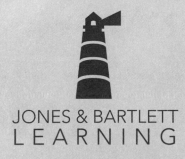

JONES & BARTLETT
LEARNING

World Headquarters
Jones & Bartlett Learning
5 Wall Street
Burlington, MA 01803
978-443-5000
info@jblearning.com
www.jblearning.com

Jones & Bartlett Learning books and products are available through most bookstores and online booksellers. To contact Jones & Bartlett Learning directly, call 800-832-0034, fax 978-443-8000, or visit our website, www.jblearning.com.

Substantial discounts on bulk quantities of Jones & Bartlett Learning publications are available to corporations, professional associations, and other qualified organizations. For details and specific discount information, contact the special sales department at Jones & Bartlett Learning via the above contact information or send an email to specialsales@jblearning.com.

Production Credits

Executive Publisher: William Brottmiller
Senior Editor: Amanda Martin
Associate Acquisitions Editor: Teresa Reilly
Editorial Assistant: Rebecca Myrick
Production Editor: Keith Henry
Senior Marketing Manager: Jennifer Stiles
VP, Manufacturing and Inventory Control: Therese Connell

Rights Clearance Editor: Amy Spencer
Composition: diacriTech
Cover Design: Kristin E. Parker
Cover Image: © Epoxy/Photodisc/Thinkstock
Printing and Binding: Edwards Brothers Malloy
Cover Printing: Edwards Brothers Malloy

To order this product, use ISBN: 978-1-284-04834-6

Library of Congress Cataloging-in-Publication Data
Heavey, Elizabeth, author.
  Statistics for nursing : a practical approach / Elizabeth Heavey.—Second edition.
    p. ; cm.
Includes bibliographical references and index.
  ISBN 978-1-284-04220-7 (pbk.)
  I. Title.
  [DNLM: 1. Statistics as Topic—Nurses' Instruction. 2. Nursing Research—methods—Nurses' Instruction. WA 950]
RT68
610.73072'7—dc23
                                                2014010416

6048

Printed in the United States of America
18 17 16 15 14   10 9 8 7 6 5 4 3 2

DEDICATION

This book is dedicated to my daughter Gabrielle, who reminds me every day how much effort, persistence, and determination it takes to try again. You have helped me be a better teacher, mother, and person just by being the brave young woman that you are. You never give up, and because of that I have watched you accomplish so much. So here is my second try at this book, and I hope it is even better than my first. I will keep trying, my beautiful girl—just like you do!

CONTENTS

CHAPTER 4: EVALUATING YOUR MEASUREMENT TOOL   49

CHAPTER 5: SAMPLING METHODS   65

CHAPTER 6: GENERATING THE RESEARCH IDEA   79

CHAPTER 7: SAMPLE SIZE, EFFECT SIZE, AND POWER   93

CHAPTER 8: CHI-SQUARE   107

CHAPTER 9: STUDENT *T*-TEST   123

CHAPTER 10: ANALYSIS OF VARIANCE (ANOVA)   143

INTRODUCTION

When the first edition of this book came out, I was very happy to hear from many nurses how useful it was in making statistics accessible for those of you just beginning to work with these concepts. You also had some very helpful suggestions, much like my own students, who provided the motivation and feedback that helped create the first edition of the book. I also heard from quite a few of you in DNP programs that the book was helpful to get you started as well, but that you also needed some introductory information about regression techniques before you could understand some of the higher level statistics texts. When I first wrote the book, DNP programs were not common, so the idea that nurses seeking clinical practice doctorates would need an introductory-level statistics text never really crossed my mind. Regression is a complicated statistical technique, so trying to introduce it in a meaningful yet understandable way was a real challenge for me. I hope you find the new chapter covering regression to be helpful.

I have acted upon the request many of you made for even more practice questions at the end of each chapter, giving you more opportunities to practice, practice, practice. I have also provided additional SPSS tutorials and article reviews on the website for the text. A few additional concepts have been added to the original chapters to create a more inclusive approach to the topic; however, I have stayed true to the original premise of the text, which is that all of this is at an introductory level without a lot of ancillary information to confuse you.

If you are teaching from this text at an undergraduate level, it is perfectly appropriate to skip the regression chapter; the rest of the content from the book will still work fine. You can also include it if it is appropriate for your students or course. As with the previous edition, the From the Statistician section examines some of the chapter concepts in greater detail.

These sections are set apart from the rest of the text and are available for students who prefer a more mathematical approach or want to have a better understanding of "why." Students who want to stick with the clinically applied information can skip these sections without experiencing problems in understanding the essential content.

The second edition of the book also includes an expanded test bank for instructors, additional multiple choice practice questions that are accessible for students and instructors alike, and additional recorded PowerPoint lectures, homework review sessions, and computer application updates. In teaching from the first edition of the book, I found that many of my students, particularly those for whom English was not a first language, appreciated and used the short recorded lectures repeatedly. It was rewarding to me to see the impact having access to this material had on their learning. Several earned the top grades in the class! With this in mind, I again opened up conversations with my students about what other tools I might be able to provide to make the material more accessible.

In talking with my students, I discovered that many are auditory learners and some are also struggling readers. Many reported that this was the first college text they read cover to cover, and they found it useful to have the limited content that was frequently repeated and applied. I was glad to hear that, but also began to wonder how I might be able to make this material more accessible so students could focus on learning the material rather than using a great deal of energy to overcome barriers to learning. So for the first time, the second edition of the book also includes an audiobook recording in which I read the essential content from the chapters (not the objectives, From the Statistician, or problems at the end). Unfortunately, the world of educational textbook publishing is not highly lucrative for authors, so I couldn't hire Brad Pitt to read the text, but I hope you find this a useful addition and can tolerate my less than perfect attempt to present the material in another useful way. My students have requested it and I have found that listening to their suggestions is always a good idea, so it is available for all of you as well. It is the same content as the chapters, so if you prefer to read the chapters go right ahead (this works better for me, a visual learner), but if you prefer to hear the chapters that option is available as well. Of course, you are welcome to use both approaches. I would suggest at least having your text with you while you listen because there are references to tables or figures, and obviously I can't read those effectively. And of course, don't forget to check the website for the book frequently for written and video tutorials, review article assignments for practice, extra practice problems and answers, and additional support options which are updated regularly.

I would love to hear from any of you who do use the new content and supports for the second edition of the text. What are your thoughts? Did these new resources help you? Do you have any other ideas for useful learning tools? Send me a quick email and help me make this material even better.

I hope you find the second edition of the book helpful and that you continue on your quest to becoming a nurse who understands statistics! You never know where it may take you someday. I certainly didn't!

All the best,
Beth

ACKNOWLEDGMENTS

This book is the product of the combined effort of many individuals who were gracious enough to contribute their time, knowledge, and effort.

Brendan Heavey is the contributing author for all of the "From the Statistician" boxes in the text. Brendan has a statistical knowledge significantly beyond my own and spent many hours writing, rewriting, and explaining concepts to make sure my simplified explanations were technically correct. I am ever grateful not only for his statistical contributions to the text, but also for his interest in and support of the project from the early proposal days. He is an incredibly gifted human being. I am proud to call him my brother.

Dr. Linda Snell, Dr. Margie Lovett-Scott, and the Department of Nursing at SUNY Brockport recognized the need for a course that explained statistics in a way that nurses could relate to and understand. They supported my efforts in developing the first class we offered and later in formalizing the material so that nurses in other locations could benefit from the curriculum.

Dr. Kathleen Peterson continues to advocate for all of us within the department and profession. She has been an incredible support both personally and professionally, and has believed in my efforts to write this second edition from the start. I consider myself to be incredibly blessed to work with such an outstanding group of individuals who make going to work a rewarding and challenging experience every day.

Jessica Jackson and Chris Passarell, both former students and now professionals working in the field, provided feedback and student perspectives, which helped me determine when I had explained a concept well and also what needed revision. Also, the many students who have taken my class throughout the years have continued to inspire me to make this edition even better and have given me lots of good ideas and perspectives that help me help you!

Many other undergraduate and graduate students emailed me from afar with feedback and thoughts about the first edition of the book. I always enjoy hearing how this book has impacted your understanding and your career, as well as your suggestions for improvement.

Thank you also to all the instructors who are using the book and letting me know how well it is working in your classrooms. You inspire and encourage me with all of your great ideas and dedication to student learning.

Thank you to the publishing team at Jones & Bartlett Learning, who saw the potential in the first edition before I did and helped make it happen, and then came back for more!

As always, my heartfelt gratitude goes to my family and friends, who loved and supported me throughout this project. I would not be where I am today without all of you. The Monday night meals, the fun family trips and college planning, the hours spent with your niece and nephew while I am away at a conference, the quiet hugs and heartfelt phone calls, the belief in me no matter what crazy plan I come up with next … I will always be grateful for each of you.

And to my children, Gabrielle and Nathaniel, you teach me every day what really matters. As I watch you grow from babies to children I am amazed by the energy, spirit, and determination you each possess. I think of you when I am teaching and remember that all of my students are another parent's pride and joy, doing their best and trying very hard. You help me be more patient, understanding, humble, and forgiving. You are the reason behind it all, my loveys. Being your Mama puts the meaning in everything that I do. I love you to the moon and the stars, to infinity and beyond and back again, forever and ever.

Thank you all.
Beth

INTRODUCTION TO STATISTICS AND LEVELS OF MEASUREMENT

HOW TO FIGURE THINGS OUT.

OBJECTIVES

By the end of this chapter students will be able to:

- State the question that statistics is always trying to answer.
- Define the empirical method.
- Compare quantitative and qualitative variables.
- Differentiate a population from a sample and a statistic from a parameter, giving an example of each.
- Explain the difference between an independent and a dependent variable, citing examples of each.

- Identify continuous and categorical variables accurately.
- Distinguish the four levels of measurement and describe each.
- Apply several beginning-level statistical techniques to further develop understanding of the concepts discussed in this chapter.

KEY TERMS

Categorical variable
A variable that has a finite number of classification groups or categories, which are usually qualitative in nature.

Continuous variable
A variable that has an infinite number of potential values, with the value being measured falling somewhere on a continuum containing in-between values.

Dependent variable
The outcome variable or final result.

Empirical method
Gathering information through systematic observation and experimentation.

Estimate
A preliminary approximation.

Independent variable
A variable measured or controlled by the experimenter; the variable that is thought to affect the outcome.

Interval data
Data whose categories are exhaustive, exclusive, and rank ordered, with equally spaced intervals.

Nominal data
Data that indicates a difference only, with categories that are exhaustive and exclusive, but not rank ordered.

Ordinal data
Data whose categories are exhaustive, exclusive, and rank ordered.

Parameter
Descriptive result for the whole group.

Population
The whole group.

Probability
How likely it is that an outcome will occur.

Qualitative measure
A measure that describes or characterizes an attribute.

Quantitative measure
A measure that reflects a numeric amount.

Ratio data
Data whose categories are exhaustive, exclusive, and rank ordered with equally spaced intervals and a point at which the variable does not exist.

Sample
A group selected from the population.

Statistic
An estimate derived from a sample.

Variable
The changing characteristic being measured.

INTRODUCTION

So here you are. You've worked hard, you are in nursing school, and are ready to begin your studies. But wait! What do you mean you have to take statistics? Why does a nurse need to understand all those numbers and equations when you just want to help people?

Most nursing students experience a mild sense of panic when they discover they have to take statistics—or any other kind of math for that matter. That reaction is commonplace. Here is a calming thought to remember: You already practice statistics, but you just don't know it.

Statistics boils down to doing two things:

- Looking at data.
- Applying tests to find out either (1) that what you observe is what you expected or (2) that your observation differs enough from what you expected that you need to change your expectations.

You might be convinced that you don't use statistics in your life, so let me give you an example. New York State, where I live, has four seasons. The summer is usually June, July, and August. Fall is September, October, and November. Winter is December, January, and February. And that leaves March, April, and May for the spring. If you walk outside in July and find it to be 80° and humid, you would draw an unspoken conclusion that what you just observed is what you were expecting, and you would put on your sunglasses. However, what if you walk outside in January and find it to be 80° and humid? You would probably be startled, take off your overcoat and boots, and read up on global warming. The difference between the weather you expect in January and what you actually encounter is so different that you might need to change your expectations. You are already practicing statistics without knowing it!

Of course, that day in January might just be a fluke occurrence (a random event), and the temperature could be below freezing again the next day. That is why we need to use the **empirical method**, otherwise known as systematic observation and experimentation. The empirical method allows you to determine whether the temperature observed is *consistently* different from what you expect. To use the empirical method, you need to check the temperature on more than one day. So you might decide to monitor the temperature for the whole

month of January to see whether readings are consistently different from what you expect. In this scenario, you would be using the empirical method to practice statistics.

POPULATION VERSUS SAMPLE

To answer questions in research, we need to set up a study of the concepts we're interested in and define multiple **variables**, that is, the changing characteristics being measured. In our example, the temperature is a variable, a measured characteristic. Each variable has an associated **probability** for each of its possible outcomes, that is, how likely it is the outcome will occur. For example, how likely is it that the temperature will be below freezing as opposed to in the eighties? In your study, you recorded the temperature for only the month of January, and those readings make up a **sample** of all the days of the year. The manner in which you collect your sample is dependent on the purpose of your study.

A sample is always a subset of a **population**, or an overall group (sometimes referred to as the reference population). In this case, our population includes all the days of the year, and the subset, or sample, is all the days in January. If you calculate the average temperature based on this sample data, you create what is called a **statistic**, which is an **estimate** generated from a sample.

A measured characteristic of a population is called a **parameter**. In our example, if you measured the temperature for the whole year and then calculated the average temperature, you would be determining a parameter. A really good way to remember the relationships among these four terms is with the following analogy: Statistic is to sample as parameter is to population.

QUANTITATIVE VERSUS QUALITATIVE

While you are collecting the weather data, you may realize that the data can be recorded in several ways. You could write down the actual temperature on that day, which would be a **quantitative measurement**, or you could describe the day as "warm" or "cold," which would be a **qualitative measurement**. A numeric amount or measure is associated with quantitative measurement (such as 80°F), and qualitative measures describe or characterize things (such as, "So darn cold I can't feel my toes").

Be careful with this difference: You can easily get confused. Qualitative variables do not contain quantity information, even if numbers are assigned. The assigned numbers have no quantitative information, rank, or distance. For example, a survey question asks, "What color scrubs are you wearing?" and lists choices numbered 1–3. Even if you selected choice 2, neon orange, you do not necessarily have any more scrubs than someone who chooses 1, lime green (although both respondents may want to purchase new scrubs). Even though these qualitative variables have numbers assigned to them, the numbers simply help with coding. The variables are still qualitative.

INDEPENDENT VERSUS DEPENDENT VARIABLES

Being as inquisitive as you are, you have probably asked yourself a number of times about a relationship you observe in your patients. For example, you notice that many supportive family members visit Sally Smith after her hip replacement recovery and that she is discharged 3 days after her surgery. Joanne Jones, on the other hand, has no visitors during her hip replacement recovery and is not discharged until day 6. As an observant nurse researcher, you have been wondering how variable x (the **independent variable**, which is measured or controlled by the experimenter) affects variable y (the **dependent variable**, or outcome variable). You wonder, does having family support (the independent variable) affect the duration of a hospital stay (the dependent, or outcome, variable)?

To answer this question, you create a study. Obviously, other factors might be involved as well, but in your experiment you are interested in how family support, the independent variable, impacts hospital stay, the dependent variable. If you are correct, then the duration of the hospital stay *depends* on family support. The independent variable can be the suspected causative agent, and the dependent variable is the measured outcome or effect.

Note: Additional criteria must be met to say a variable is causative, so I refer here only to the "suspected" causative agent.

CONTINUOUS VERSUS CATEGORICAL VARIABLES

Some data have an infinite number of potential values, and the value you measure falls somewhere on a continuum containing in-between values. These values are called **continuous variables**. As a nurse, when you measure your patient's temperature, you are measuring a continuous variable. The reading could be 98° or 98.6° or 98.66666°. The infinite possibilities are all quantitative in nature. Actually, the only limit to the measurement is the accuracy of the measuring device. If, for example, you have a thermometer that measures only

FROM THE STATISTICIAN *Brendan Heavey*

What is a Statistic?

As a student of statistics, you will run into questions regarding parameters and statistics all the time. Determining the difference between the two can be difficult. To get a concrete idea of the difference, let's look at an example. According to the Bureau of Labor Statistics, registered nurses constitute the largest healthcare occupation, with 2.7 million jobs nationwide. Because this text is primarily designed for nursing students, let's use this number for our example.

Let's say you are a consultant working for a fledgling company that is planning to make scrubs for nurses. Let's call this company Carol's Nursing Scrubs, Inc. Scrubs at Carol's will come in small, medium, and large. The company will offer all kinds of styles and prints, but the underlying sizes are intended to remain the same. Carol just received her first bit of seed money to mass-produce 20,000 pairs of scrubs. Carol, an overly demanding boss, wants the medium-size scrubs to fit as many nurses nationwide as possible. To make that happen, she needs to know the average height and weight of nurses nationwide, so she has instructed you to conduct a nationwide poll. She thinks you should ask every nurse in the country his or her height and weight and then calculate the average of all the numbers you get.

Now, you are an intelligent, well-grounded employee who's in demand everywhere and working for Carol only because her health plan comes with a sweet gym membership and you get a company car. So you realize it would be pretty difficult to set up a nationwide poll and ask all the nurses in the country for their height and weight. Even if you tried a mass mailing, the data returned to you would be filled with so many incompletes and errors that it wouldn't be trustworthy.

So what are you to do? Your first instinct might be to respond to your boss by saying, "Geez, Carol, that's so absurd and impossible I don't even know where I'd start," and then finish your day on the golf range. However, after this course you'll be not only a nurse, but a nurse with some training in statistics. You'll be able to deal with this situation in a more effective way.

Jenna the Statistical Nursing Guru (you):	Carol, I recommend we take a few *samples* of nurses nationwide and *survey* them rather than attempting to contact every nurse in the country. Then we could *estimate* the true average height and weight based on our samples.
Carol:	How would that work, Jenna?
Jenna:	Well, I'd go down to the University Hospital and poll 30 RNs on their height and weight. Then I'd go to the next state and do the same. My third and final sample would contain 30 RNs from a hospital in Springfield. I'd calculate the average from my total *sample* (90 RNs), which is a *statistic,* and use that to estimate the overall average in the United States, which is a *parameter* of the total *population*. You see, Carol, any time you calculate an estimate with data from a sample or list the data from the sample itself, you calculate a statistic. If you calculate an estimate from data in an entire population, you're calculating a parameter.

in whole degrees, you will not have as much information as you would using a thermometer that measures to the one-thousandth of a degree.

Continuous variables can be contrasted with **categorical variables**, sometimes called discrete variables, which have a finite number of classification groups, or categories, that are usually qualitative in nature. For example, as part of your research you may need to collect information about your patients' racial background. The choices available are African American, Native American, Caucasian, Asian, Latino, mixed race, and other. Race is an example of a categorical variable, a measurement that is restricted to a specific value and does not have any fractional or in-between values.

LEVELS OF MEASUREMENT

Let's say your interest in the relationship between family support (the independent variable) and duration of stay (the dependent variable) is extensive enough that you apply for a program at your hospital that includes a small research fellowship. You win the fellowship and proceed to collect data about each patient admitted to your orthopedic unit for hip replacement over a 3-month period. The study protocol calls for you to complete the usual admission forms and then for patients to complete a short survey about perceived family support. After your institutional review board approves your study, you begin. The level of measurement of your data determines what type of analysis you are able to perform in your study, so let's look at the different types and what makes each level unique.

Your first question asks the patient's gender: male or female. The data you gather for this question is an example of **nominal data**; it simply indicates a difference between the two answers. One is neither greater nor less than the other, and they are not in any particular order. Also, the categories are exclusive and exhaustive; that is, the patient cannot answer "both" or "neither."

You then ask the patient to rate his or her family support level as low, medium, or high. This question is an example of **ordinal data**. Ordinal data must be exhaustive and exclusive, just like nominal data, but the answers are also rank ordered. With rank-ordered data, each observation/category is higher or lower or better or worse than another, but you do not know the level of difference between the observations/categories. In this example, a high level of family support indicates a greater quantity of the variable in question than does a low level of family support.

A routine part of admitting each patient also includes a baseline set of vital signs. One of the vital signs you check is each patient's temperature. Temperature is an example of **interval data**, which is exhaustive, exclusive, and rank ordered and which has numerically equal intervals. In this example, the interval is a degree of Fahrenheit.

After assessing each patient's temperature, you go on to take each patient's blood pressure. Blood pressure is an example of **ratio data**, which is exhaustive, exclusive, and rank ordered with equal intervals *and* a point at which the variable is absent. (If the blood pressure reading is "absent" in any of your patients, you need to begin CPR!)

Ratio data is the highest level of measurement you can collect and gives you the greatest number of options for data analysis, but not all variables can be measured at this level. As a general rule of thumb, always collect the highest-level data you can for all your variables, especially your dependent variable. In your study of how family support (the independent variable) impacts the duration of hospital stay (the dependent variable), you could have measured the length of hospital stay as short, medium, or long (ordinal) or in actual days (the interval/ratio level). Obviously, the actual number of days gives you a higher level of measurement.

Note: A dependent variable with a higher level of measurement allows for a more robust data analysis. Collect the highest level you can.

SUMMARY

Talk about exhausting, but you survived! So let's wrap it up here. Statistics really boils down to asking:

- Is what you observe what you expect?
- Or, using the empirical method, have you determined that what you observe is different enough from what you would expect that you need to change your expectations?

Using qualitative (descriptive) and quantitative (numeric) variables, you can assess the impact of independent variables on dependent (outcome) variables. Always collect the highest level of measurement possible, especially for your dependent variable. Doing so gives you the widest range of analysis options when you are ready to "crunch the numbers."

If you understand these concepts, you are ready to move on to the review exercises. If you are still struggling, don't despair. These concepts sometimes take a while to absorb. Read the review questions and then the chapter again, and slowly start to look at the review questions. You will get the hang of statistics; sometimes you just need practice. My students frequently look at me as though I am an alien when I tell them that by the end of the course this chapter will seem really simple. You may not believe it either. However, as you develop your understanding and apply these concepts, they will become clearer, and you too will look back in amazement. You are a statistical genius in the making!

CHAPTER 1 REVIEW QUESTIONS

1. A researcher asks hospitalized individuals about their comfort in a new type of hospital gown. This is an example of what type of data?

   a. ratio
   b. independent
   c. quantitative
   d. qualitative

2. If a researcher is examining how exposure to cigarette ads affects smoking behavior, cigarette ads are what type of variable?

   a. qualitative
   b. quantitative
   c. dependent
   d. independent

3. A nurse practitioner measures how many times per minute a heart beats when an individual is at rest versus when running. She is measuring the heartbeat at what level of measurement?

   a. interval/ratio
   b. nominal
   c. independent
   d. ordinal

4. If a researcher is examining how exposure to cigarette ads affects smoking behavior, smoking behavior is what type of variable?

    a. ratio
    b. independent
    c. dependent
    d. nominal

5. The research nurse is coding adults according to size. A person with a below-average body mass index (BMI) is coded as 1, average is 2, and above-average is 3. What level of measurement is this?

    a. nominal
    b. ratio
    c. ordinal
    d. interval

6. You are asked to design a study measuring how nutritional status is related to serum lead levels in children. You assess calcium and fat intake, as well as serum lead levels in a sample of 30 children who are 2 years old. Lead levels are measured in micrograms per deciliter (mcg/dL). One child had a lead level of 17 mcg/dL. This is an example of what type of variable?

    a. quantitative
    b. qualitative
    c. independent
    d. nominal

Questions 7–9: You are asked to design a study to examine the relationship between preoperative blood pressure and postoperative hematocrit.

7. What is your independent variable?

_____

8. What is your dependent variable?

_____

9. How will you measure each, and what level of measurement is this?

_____

_____

Questions 10–13: You are later asked to do a follow-up study to see whether requiring an intraoperative blood transfusion impacted postoperative rates of poor mental health, specifically depression.

10. What is your independent variable?

_____

11. What is your dependent variable?

_____

12. How will you measure them and why?

_____

_____

13. Is your dependent variable measured at the highest level? If not, why not?

_____

_____

Questions 14–16: You decide to measure depression on the following scale: 1 = low, 2 = moderate, 3 = high.

14. What level of measurement is this?

15. How could this measure be improved?

16. Why might you want to improve it?

17. You decide to measure postoperative hematocrit by serum levels. Is this a quantitative or qualitative measurement?

18. You discover that all but those with the lowest hematocrits had higher levels of depression after their surgery and transfusion. Why might the group that had the most critical need for the transfusions not have the subsequent depression associated with this result in the rest of your sample?

Questions 19–25: Elevated serum lead levels in childhood are associated with lower IQ, hyperactivity, aggression, poor growth, diminished academic performance, increased delinquency, seizures, and even death. The neurological damage that occurs cannot be reversed, even once exposure is stopped.

19. You have been asked to follow up in your community and determine what outcomes are associated with lead exposure in children. List three dependent variables for your study and how you will measure them.

20. What level of measurement are your dependent variables? Are they continuous or categorical?

21. Can you increase the level of measurement for any of them?

22. If you are looking at what outcomes are associated with lead exposure in children, what is your independent variable?

23. Why might it be difficult to measure?

24. Describe how it could be measured quantitatively or qualitatively.

_____

_____

25. Which do you prefer? Why?

_____

_____

Questions 26–34: A nurse researcher is assessing how well patients respond to two different dosing regimens of a new drug approved to treat diabetic neuropathy. Two different dosing regimens are administered and side effects are monitored. Results are shown in Figure 1-1.

26. What is the independent variable?

_____

27. What are the dependent variables?

_____

28. In this study, the nurse researcher measures the side effects as present or not present. This variable is what level of measurement?

_____

29. If instead, the nurse researcher decided to measure weight gain in pounds gained, what level of measurement would it be? Would it be a continuous or categorical variable?

_____

FIGURE 1-1   **Self-Reported Side Effects of Two Randomized Groups of 100 Individuals Treated for Diabetic Neuropathy.**

Side Effect Reported	Low Dosage	High Dosage
Nausea	8	21
Headache	3	5
Weight gain	1	0
Weight loss	0	6
Lethargy	3	11
Skin rash	13	13

30. If she decided to measure nausea as present, limiting, or debilitating, what level of measurement would it be? Would nausea be a continuous or categorical variable?

---

31. If she measured nausea as the number of hours of nausea experienced in a day, what level of measurement would it be?

---

32. If the nurse researcher asked the subjects to describe their headache, would this be a quantitative or a qualitative variable? In the second phase of this study, the nurse researcher asks the study participants to report changes in signs and symptoms of their neuropathy. She determines that those on the low-dose regimen had a similar level of pain relief and improvement in mobility as those who took the high-dose drug regimen.

---

33. What is the dependent variable in the second phase of the study?

---

34. Considering the information you now know about the side effects and relief of neuropathy symptoms, what might you prefer as a patient and why? What else might you want to know before making the decision?

ANSWERS TO CHAPTER 1 REVIEW QUESTIONS

1. D

3. A

5. C

7. Preoperative blood pressure

9. Answers may vary—actual blood pressure ratio, lab-reported hematocrit ratio, and so on.

11. Depression

13. Answers may vary.

15. Use of interval data, such as Beck's depression scale

17. Quantitative

19. Answers may vary, including IQ, school enrollment, crime, pregnancy, hematocrit, learning disabilities, growth, hearing, and behavior.

21. Answers will vary.

23. Answers may vary, and include, "It requires a blood draw," "There are different testing mechanisms," "The level may change depending on when the exposure occurred and the time that has lapsed since then," "Levels may differ from fingersticks versus serum draws."

25. Answers will vary.

27. Side effects, nausea, headache, weight gain, weight loss, lethargy, skin rash

29. Ratio, continuous

31. Ratio

33. Signs and symptoms of neuropathy

CHAPTER 2

PRESENTING DATA

WILL MY AUDIENCE BE ABLE TO SEE WHAT THE DATA IS SAYING?

By the end of this chapter students will be able to:

- Describe a frequency distribution.
- Calculate the cumulative frequency and the cumulative percentages for a group of data.
- Identify situations in which a grouped frequency distribution is helpful.

- Develop a frequency distribution.
- Calculate a percentage.
- Identify the best visual representation for various types of data.
- Determine the percentile rank of an observation.

KEY TERMS

Bar Chart
A chart that has the nominal variable on the horizontal axis and the frequency of the response on the vertical axis, with spaces between the bars on the horizontal axis.

Cumulative frequency
The number of observations with a value less than the maximum value of the variable interval.

Cumulative percentage
The percentage of observations with a value less than the maximum value of the variable interval.

Cumulative relative frequency
Calculated by adding together all the relative frequencies less than or equal to the selected upper limit point.

Frequency distribution
A summary of the numerical counts of the values or categories of a measurement.

Grouped frequency
A frequency distribution with distinct intervals or groups created to simplify the information.

Histogram
A chart that usually has an ordinal variable on the horizontal axis and the frequency of the response on the vertical axis, with no spaces between the columns on the horizontal axis.

Line graph
A chart in which the horizontal axis shows the passage of time and the vertical axis marks the value of the variable at that particular time.

Outlier
An extreme value of a variable, outside the expected range.

Percentage
A portion of the whole.

Percentile rank
The percentage of observations below a particular value.

Percentiles
Divide the data set into 100 equal portions.

Quartiles
Divide the data set into four equal portions, with the first quartile being the 25th percentile, the second quartile being the 50th percentile, and the third quartile being the 75th percentile.

Relative frequency
The number of times a particular observation occurs divided by the total number of observations.

Scatterplot
A chart in which each point represents the measurement of one subject in terms of two variables.

FREQUENCY DISTRIBUTIONS

Once you have designed a study and collected data, the next step is to decide how to present the assembled data. You have several options for doing so. The first and most common choice is a **frequency distribution**, which shows the frequency of each measure of a variable. A frequency distribution is created by gathering all the responses collected from a sample of variables into a table (see **Figure 2-1**). The first column of the

| FIGURE 2-1 | Frequency Distribution Table for the Length of the Hospital Stay. |

Days Spent in the Hospital Postop	Number of Patients Who Stayed This Long (Frequency)	Number of Patients Who Stayed This Long or Less (Cumulative Frequency)
0	0	0
1	0	0
2	2	2
3	7	9
4	23	32
5	14	46
6	4	50

frequency distribution in Figure 2-1 shows the number of days spent postoperatively in the hospital (the dependent variable), sorted from the shortest stay to the longest. The second column shows how frequently that length of stay was needed, that is, the number of patients who spent each number of post-operative days in the hospital. These two columns display the total numeric value of the variable of interest (in this case, the dependent variable, days spent in the hospital), usually ordered from the lowest to the highest. You can see the frequency of each level of the variable and its spread (distribution).

Sometimes it is also helpful to include the **relative frequency** of an observation, which is just the number of times a particular observation occurs divided by the total number of observations. For example, according to Figure 2-1, seven patients stayed in the hospital for 3 days. If you wanted to report the relative frequency of staying 3 days, you would divide the number of patients who stayed for 3 days by the total number of patients included in the study; in this example, that would be 7 divided by 50, or a relative frequency of 14%. Relative frequency is a helpful concept to illustrate what proportion of the observations this particular observation is. The frequency distribution table presents a big-picture view of your data.

To augment a frequency distribution table and really impress your colleagues, you can add a **cumulative frequency** column, which simply lists the number of observations with a value less than the maximum value of the variable interval. For example, in the third column of Figure 2-1, in the second row, the number 9 means that nine patients have stayed either 0, 1, 2, or 3 days postop in the hospital. The number 9 is the cumulative frequency for the first four intervals (0, 1, 2, and

3 days) of the variable. Let's say you are putting together an in-service presentation and decide to collect data from a set of patients on how many postop days they spent in the hospital. You find that nine patients were discharged on day 3 or earlier; that total includes all the patients who stayed for 0, 1, 2, or 3 days. It is a cumulative frequency. You may also want to report a **cumulative relative frequency**, which just totals the relative frequencies up to the upper limit point you have selected. In this example, if you wanted to report the cumulative relative frequency for staying 3 days or less, you would simply add up the relative frequencies for those staying 0, 1, 2, and 3 days ($0/50 + 0/50 + 2/50 + 7/50 = 9/50$ or 0.18 or 18%). This can be helpful when presenting your report because most individuals can understand percentages fairly well.

Now your nurse manager approaches you in a panic because the accreditation agency is coming next week and she needs to know how many patients were discharged after more than 4 days of recovery. The best way to visually answer that question is to create a new table that includes **grouped frequencies**, which is a frequency distribution with distinct intervals or groups created to simplify the information. In **Figure 2-2**, the values of the frequency distribution in Figure 2-1 have been collected into two groups: (1) patients who spent 4 days or fewer in postop and (2) those who spent 5 days or more. Grouped frequencies are typically used when working with a lot of data and an entire frequency distribution is simply too large to be meaningful.

Unfortunately, when data is grouped, some information is lost. For example, how many patients in Figure 2-2 stayed for only 2 days? The answer is not discernible from this table. This is the first drawback to be aware of when using grouped frequencies; you can lose a lot of information when you convert your data into groups, especially if you use large intervals. You can even make the intervals so large that they are meaningless. In our example, if one interval were more than 7 days and the other were less than 7 days, the table in Figure 2-2 would not be very useful anymore because all the patients in the study were discharged by day 7. On the other hand, make sure not to make the intervals too small or your grouped frequency won't have any benefit over a standard frequency distribution.

Let's return to our example of the poor nurse manager who needed to get ready for the accreditation agency visit. After retabulating

FIGURE 2-2	**Frequency Distribution Table for the Length of Hospital Stay Using Grouped Frequencies.**

Days Spent in the Hospital Postop	Number of Patients Who Stayed This Long (Frequency)
≤ 4 days	32
5 or more days	18

the data as shown in Figure 2-2, you can calmly go into her office and tell her that, during the period of time in your study, 18 patients were discharged after more than 4 days of recovery.

PERCENTAGES

A **percentage** is a part of the whole. To calculate a percentage, divide the partial number of items by the total number of items and then multiply that quantity by 100. For example, what if that same nurse manager asked you, "What percentage of our patients do those 18 represent?" You could do the simple calculation shown in **Figure 2-3**. In this example, the number of patients of interest (those who were discharged after day 4) is 18. The total number of patients studied is 50. (See the last line of the third column in Figure 2-1.) The first step in our calculation is 18 divided by 50. This division results in 0.36, which is then multiplied by 100 to get a percentage of 36%.

Exam scores are a classic example of percentages. If you take an exam with 30 questions and get 27 correct, what is your overall score? In this case, divide 27 by 30 and then multiply by 100 to get 90%.

A statistics concept commonly associated with percentages is **cumulative percentage**, which is the percentage of observations with a value less than the maximum value of the variable interval. The idea is the same as cumulative frequency, but expressed as a percentage. See the rightmost column of the table in **Figure 2-4** for an example. The last column shows the conversion of each cumulative frequency (from Figure 2-1) into a cumulative percentage.

| FIGURE 2-3 | **Calculating a Percentage.** |

$$\frac{18}{50} = 0.36 \times 100 = 36\%$$

| FIGURE 2-4 | **Cumulative Percentage Table for Length of Hospital Stay.** |

Days Spent in the Hospital Postop	Number of Patients Who Stayed This Long	Cumulative Frequency	Cumulative Percentage
0	0	0	$0/50 = 0 \times 100 = 0\%$
1	0	0	$0/50 = 0 \times 100 = 0\%$
2	2	2	$2/50 = 0.04 \times 100 = 4\%$
3	7	9	$9/50 = 0.18 \times 100 = 18\%$
4	23	32	$32/50 = 0.64 \times 100 = 64\%$
5	14	46	$46/50 = 0.92 \times 100 = 92\%$
6	4	50	$50/50 = 1.0 \times 100 = 100\%$

That column shows what percentage of patients had a hospital stay of less than or equal to the number of days listed in that row. For example, 18% of patients had a hospital stay of less than or equal to 3 days, and all of the patients (100%) were discharged on or before day 6 (see the last line of the last column).

Percentages are also closely related to percentiles, which are explained in the next "From the Statistician."

From the Statistician *Brendan Heavey*

Quantiles, Quartiles, and Percentiles—Oh My!

The terms "quantiles," "quartiles," and "percentiles" cause a lot of people grief because they are so closely related. So let's break them down a little. Using quantiles is just like dividing a data set into different portions or bins. Two special cases of quantiles are percentiles and quartiles.

- **Percentiles** divide a data set into 100 equal portions. You see this concept used with body mass index (BMI). If a patient's BMI is in the 90th percentile, then 90% of the BMIs in the reference population used to develop the distribution were at or below this patient's BMI. Put another way, this patient's BMI is in the top 10% of the reference population.
- **Quartiles** divide a data set into four equal parts. For example, suppose your nursing manager wants to hire only students who finished in the top quarter of the class on a particular exam. She would calculate the third quartile and select all the scores above it. Because your score would clearly be near the top, she would then rush to your school and attempt to woo you with new scrubs and tuition benefits!

How would the nursing manager compute a percentile? Let's say a sample of 331 nurses at Massachusetts General Hospital were asked how many patients they see on average each shift. The results of this survey are shown in **Figure 2-5**. A nice formula to find percentiles in the ordered data set is shown in **Figure 2-6**. For instance, based on the ordered data set in Table 2-5, we apply the formula as shown in **Figure 2-7** to find what is called the median, or the middle observation when the observations are lined up in rank order (least to greatest). The median is also the 50th percentile. Therefore, our median is our 166th observation. Using Figure 2-5, we can see that the nurse who was observation #166 saw 16 patients.

Because the total sample is 331, the middle observation is the 166th observation. If you add all the nurses who saw fewer than 16 patients, you find that 155 of them reported seeing fewer than 16 patients and 22 others saw 16 patients. After lining up the observations in rank order, the 166th observation falls into the group who reported seeing 16 patients; that group is the median. Using the formula takes less time than the old-fashioned way: adding them up.

You can also check yourself by looking at the cumulative relative frequency column. The median should be where the midpoint is. In Figure 2-5, look at the row for 15 patients, and see the corresponding cumulative frequency percentage; 47% of the nurses reported seeing 15 or fewer patients. Look at the next line, for 16 patients; 53% of the nurses reported seeing 16 or fewer patients. Therefore, the 50th percentile is above 15 and less than or equal to 16. Because we cannot split a patient into parts (at least for statistical purposes!), the median number of patients is 16.

FIGURE 2-5   **Frequency Table for a Sample of 331 Nurses at Massachusetts General Hospital.**

Number of Patients	Number of Nurses	Relative Frequency (%)	Cumulative Relative Frequency (%)	Number of Patients	Number of Nurses	Relative Frequency (%)	Cumulative Relative Frequency (%)
1	0	0	0	16	22	7	53
2	0	0	0	17	20	6	60
3	2	1	1	18	19	6	65
4	3	1	2	19	18	5	71
5	5	2	3	20	19	6	76
6	8	2	5	21	17	5	82
7	8	2	8	22	15	5	86
8	9	3	11	23	12	4	90
9	9	3	13	24	8	2	92
10	12	4	17	25	9	3	95
11	14	4	21	26	5	2	96
12	18	5	27	27	5	2	98
13	22	7	33	28	3	1	99
14	23	7	40	29	3	1	100
15	22	7	47	30	1	0	100

Three hundred and thirty-one nurses at Massachusetts General Hospital were asked how many patients they saw on their shifts that night. Results are displayed. Relative frequencies are computed by dividing the number of nurses who saw each number of patients by the total number of nurses (331). Each cumulative relative frequency is the result of adding the previous row's relative frequency to its cumulative relative frequency, so in essence, cumulative relative frequency is an accumulation of relative frequency.

FIGURE 2-6   **Formula for Calculating Percentiles in an Ordered Data Set.**

$$P_{obs}^{th} = (n+1) \times \frac{y}{100}$$

where

P_{obs}^{th} = The number of the observations at the percentile for which you are looking

n = The number of observations in your data set

y = The percentile you're looking for

FIGURE 2-7   **Equation for the Massachusetts General Sample.**

$$P_{abs}^{th} = (331 + 1) \times \frac{50}{100} = 166$$

Percentages are also related to the concept of the **percentile rank** of a score, which is the percentage of observations lower than that score in a frequency distribution. For example, if your test score is greater than 75% of all the scores for the class, it is at the 75th percentile.

BAR CHARTS

Remember nominal categorical data (the categorical data that shows only a difference and is not rank ordered)? A **bar chart** is one way to display this type of data. A common way to set up the bar chart is to line up the responses for the nominal variable along the horizontal axis and place the frequencies of the responses on the vertical axis. Bar charts are typically used for nominal categorical data with spaces between the bars because each answer is distinct and in no particular order. For example, if you collected data about the marital status of fellow nurses on your unit, you might find data like in **Figure 2-8**. A quick look at the bar chart makes it apparent that there are more of the nurses working on this unit who are single than either married or other. The bar chart gives you a good visual representation of nominal categorical data.

Bar charts can be used for ordinal data as well, but then the bars should follow the rank order of the variable categories.

FIGURE 2-8   **Bar Chart for Marital Status.**

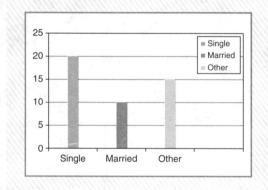

HISTOGRAMS

Histograms are a type of bar chart. Histograms often have no spaces between the bars because these charts are most frequently used to display either ordinal data or continuous data. (Remember, ordinal data has categories that show a ranked difference; continuous data has an infinite number of possible in-between measures.) For example, pain may be rated as mild, moderate, or severe.

Presenting these types of data in a histogram shows how frequently each response is selected and allows for visual comparison of the different levels. In **Figure 2-9**, 11 patients were interviewed 12 hours postop from abdominal surgery. Six rated their pain as severe, four stated it was moderate,

FIGURE 2-9 **Histogram for Pain Level.**

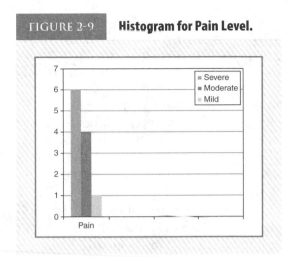

FIGURE 2-10 **Line Graph for Length of Hospitalization.**

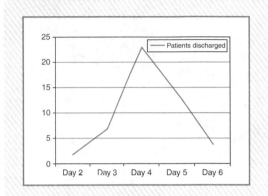

and one felt it was only mild (she had just had her pain meds). The lack of spaces between the bars in the histogram reinforces the idea that these responses are on a continuum and that the order is illustrated on that continuum.

Looking at this histogram gives you a big-picture idea of the pain these patients experienced. In this case, the histogram seems to indicate that many postop patients report the first 24 hours as being very painful. So the next time you orient a new nurse, you might remember to point out how important it is to make sure patients have their pain medicine ordered and administered on time immediately after surgery. The chart also visually displays that many patients may not be getting adequate pain medication because so many report severe pain. After collecting this data, you may decide to review the unit protocols for pain management.

LINE GRAPHS

Continuous variables that change over time are frequently best illustrated in a **line graph**. The horizontal axis shows the passage of time, and the vertical axis marks the value of the variable over time. For example, the data from the cumulative frequency example about days of hospitalization is illustrated in **Figure 2-10**. The chart shows that most of the patients needed to stay 4 days postop before going home. You might want to compare this line graph to another after you institute an early mobilization plan with your surgical patients to see whether the length of hospitalization has changed.

SCATTERPLOTS

Scatterplots are a little different from the previously discussed graphs in that each point represents how one subject relates to two variables. For example, **Figure 2-11** shows a scatterplot of height in inches and weight in pounds for a group of eight kindergartners. Each square on the scatterplot represents one student. The horizontal axis displays that student's height, and the vertical axis displays his or her weight. You can see from the direction

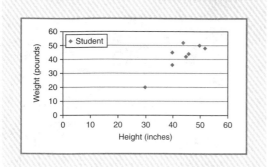

FIGURE 2-11 **Scatterplot for Student Height (x axis) and Weight (y axis).**

student who is only 30 inches and 20 pounds clearly stands out from the rest of the group. Perhaps the child is just extremely small, or there may have been an error in measurement, recording, or data entry. If there are a lot of outliers, a nurse may decide either that further investigation is needed to ensure accuracy or that the outliers may actually represent the children the study is designed to identify. One example of this technique is the use of growth charts. In almost all cases when children make pediatric visits, nurses plot the children's heights and weights on a growth chart. This is one example of using a scatterplot to look for outliers. If a child isn't growing properly, recognizing the growth pattern as an outlier is one way to identify a child who needs intervention.

of the plotted points that as students get taller, they usually get heavier as well; that's the relationship between the two variables. When points are close together or seem to follow a line closely, the relationship between the variables on the horizontal and vertical axes are relatively strong.

When you look at a scatterplot, note the general trend. In this example, the plotted points start low on the left side and move up as they progress toward the right side. This pattern indicates a *positive relationship* between height and weight (in other words, they usually move in the same direction—when height increases, weight usually does too). If the plotted points were to start in the upper left corner and slope down to the right, the pattern would indicate a *negative relationship* between the two variables (such as exercise and weight—when exercise is increased, weight usually decreases).

Scatterplots also give nurses a chance to look for **outliers**, or data that is outside the expected relationship. In Figure 2-11, the

SUMMARY

This chapter contained quite a bit of information, so let's review and make sure you are really comfortable with it. Frequently, researchers put a great deal of time into collecting data and very little time into thinking about how to present it; however, how you present your data often determines whether your intended audience understands your work or is even interested in it. (Teachers are all aware of this point!) The most common choice for presentations is a frequency distribution, which shows the frequency of each measure of a variable. You can add up these frequencies and create either cumulative frequency columns or grouped frequencies, depending on the question you are trying to answer.

You can also calculate percentages, which are parts of the whole. Because many nurses are familiar with them, percentages are sometimes a useful way to convey information. You can then add up the percentages and present a cumulative percentage, which is simply the percentage of observations with a value less than the maximum value of the interval.

Another way to convey information is with a visual graph, such as a bar chart for nominal data, a histogram for ordinal or continuous data, a line graph for continuous variables that change over time, or a scatterplot in which one subject's values for two variables are graphed. You need to decide which type of chart will work the best for the audience you are trying to reach. Just remember, use color, make it bigger, avoid just using lots and lots of numbers in a row—and bring coffee because most nurses are considerably sleep deprived!

CHAPTER 2 REVIEW QUESTIONS

1. A study of 30 fathers was completed in which the fathers were asked the highest level of education they had completed. Ten completed only elementary school; 10 completed elementary and high school; 7 completed elementary, high school, and college; and 3 completed elementary, high school, college, and graduate school. What was the cumulative percentage of fathers who completed only elementary school? Round to the nearest whole number.

2. In your study of 40 people, 8 had no cold symptoms, 12 had mild cold symptoms, 9 had moderate cold symptoms, and 10 had severe cold symptoms. One patient was lost to follow-up and no data could be collected. What percentage of patients reported cold symptoms?

3. Given the information in question 2, what percentage of patients reported no cold symptoms?

4. Use the frequency distribution in **Figure 2-12** to construct a bar chart for influenza cases in your hospital during 8 months of 2013. How would your chart look different if it were a histogram? Discuss at least one rationale for selecting either a bar chart or a histogram to present this data.

Questions 5–7: Your community begins a large-scale influenza vaccine effort, and the following year the number of cases drops (see **Figure 2-13**).

5. Construct a line graph showing the data from 2013 and the data from 2014. Compare the two.

| FIGURE 2-12 | **Influenza Cases for 2013.** |

Month	Number of Cases
August	18
September	29
October	68
November	107
December	158
January	166
February	160
March	111

| FIGURE 2-13 | **Influenza Cases for 2014.** |

Month	Number of Cases
August	19
September	27
October	31
November	34
December	48
January	59
February	51
March	45

6. Why didn't the numbers change significantly for August and September?

_____

7. Do you consider the vaccine effort to be successful? Why?

_____
_____

Research Application

Questions 8–13: See the data in **Figure 2-14**.

8. Construct a bar chart for mother's marital status.

9. What percentage of the adolescents are employed? What percentage of the adolescents are in school? Are these variables quantitative or qualitative? Round to the nearest tenth of a percent.

_____
_____
_____

10. Identify the level of measurement of each variable.

_____
_____
_____

FIGURE 2-14   **Demographic Characteristics of 92 Adolescents Completing a Family Planning Survey.**

	n (%)
Pregnancy status	
Pregnant	78 (84.7)
Not Pregnant	14 (15.2)
Age	
≤ 14 years old	2 (2.2)
15–17 years old	46 (50)
18–19 years old	43 (46.7)
Number in household*	
< 6 people	70 (79.5)
≥ 6 people	18 (20.5)
Student status†	
Not in school	46 (50.5)
In school	45 (49.4)
Mother's marital status	
Single	38 (41.3)
Married	27 (29.3)
Divorced	13 (14.1)
Other	14 (15.2)
Employment status	
Employed	25 (27.2)
Not employed	67 (72.8)

*Missing *n* = 4
†Missing *n* = 1

11. Could any of these variables have been measured as continuous quantitative variables?

12. Construct a histogram for the ages of the adolescents. Describe the histogram's shape and what it tells you about this sample population. Why would a histogram be an appropriate choice for presenting this data?

_____

_____

13. Is the pregnancy status of this group of adolescents typical? Why might that be?

_____

_____

14. You've been recruited by the head of the Federal Emergency Management Agency (FEMA) to act as the head triage nurse for a large city's hurricane response team. One of your main duties is to decide which nurses will cover which facilities in the overall relief effort. Because most nursing duties will have to change during this shift in personnel, you decide to divide the group based on years of experience. Your nurse's aide carries out a brief survey of all the personnel available (100 nurses) and gives you a list of number of years of experience for each (see **Figure 2-15**). Find the quartiles of this distribution, and assign a role to each nurse. For example, the nurses with the least amount of experience should be assigned to the rescue team, and the ones with the most experience should be assigned to the intensive care unit (ICU).

_____

_____

| FIGURE 2-15 | **Nurses Available for the Hurricane Response Team.** |

Number of Years' Experience	Number of Nurses	Number of Years' Experience	Number of Nurses
2	15	12	3
3	10	13	3
4	9	15	3
5	8	18	3
6	8	20	2
7	9	25	2
8	6	32	1
9	5	35	1
10	5	36	1
11	5	40	1

Coordinated Hurricane Response

| Rescue Team | Stadium | Hospital | ICU |

Questions 15–18: A diabetes educator is working with a group of 15 patients who have been newly diagnosed with type 2 diabetes. She administers a brief pretest, reviews carbohydrate counting with them, and then asks them to complete a posttest assessing their knowledge of the total grams of carbohydrate found in one serving of four sample items brought to the class. The results are shown in **Figure 2-16**.

15. Complete the Cumulative Frequency column of the table.

16. What percentage of the patients answered all four questions correctly?

17. Add another column to the table and calculate the cumulative percentage.

18. The diabetes educator would like you to present her results in a grouped frequency table showing the frequency and percentage of those who passed the posttest with > 70% and those who didn't for the report she has to make to her funding agency. Show your product.

Questions 19–20: A researcher examining patients diagnosed with sarcoidosis would like to look at trends in their inflammatory markers. The researcher would like to use a graph that can illustrate the erythrocyte sedimentation rate and the C-reactive protein level for each individual in the study to visually illustrate the relationship between the two markers.

19. What graphic representation of the data would you suggest?

20. After creating this graph, the researcher notices one of the subjects is significantly below the trend line the other subjects seem to follow. What might be a logical explanation for this outlier?

FIGURE 2-16   Posttest Assessing Carbohydrate Knowledge.

Number Correct on the Posttest	Number of Patients Who Answered This Number of Questions Correctly (Frequency)	Number Who Answered This Many or Fewer Questions Correctly (Cumulative Frequency)
0	1	
1	1	
2	2	
3	6	
4	5	

21. An emergency room nurse working in a hospital in the wine region of the Finger Lakes in New York has noticed a seasonal trend for ocular injuries from bottle corks. She would like to illustrate this graphically and develops a histogram. Why might she prefer a histogram to a bar chart?

_____

22. When the nurse looks at her data and the histogram it is apparent that more ocular injuries from bottle corks occur in October (which is wine fermentation season) and January. She also notices that more of the injuries involve the right eye. Provide a reasonable explanation for both the January peak and the prevalence of the right eye injuries.

_____

23. The nurse would like to determine if more ocular injuries are associated with wine bottles from Sharespeak winery or from bottles from Francesco's winery. What would be the independent variable?

_____

24. What would be the dependent variable?

_____

25. You are tracking melanoma in your county. Calculate the race- and gender-specific mortality rates from the data provided in **Figure 2-17**.

| FIGURE 2-17 | **Melanoma Data.** |

	New Cases	**Deaths**	**Population**	**Mortality Rate**
Men	5	2	25,000	
Women	3	1	25,000	
White	7	3	40,000	
African American	1	0	10,000	

26. Offer a potential explanation for why the race-specific rates may be different for whites and African Americans.

_____

ANSWERS TO CHAPTER 2 REVIEW QUESTIONS

1. 33%

3. 20%

5. Answer includes line graph; beginning in October there is a substantial decrease in cases.

7. Yes, there was a substantial decrease in cases beginning in October after the vaccine was administered.

9. 27.2%, 49.4%, qualitative

11. Yes, age, number in household, years in school, years employed

13. No, all of the adolescents were waiting for pregnancy or family planning—related services.

15.

Number Correct on the Posttest	Number of Patients Who Answered This Number of Questions Correctly (Frequency)	Number Who Answered This Many or Fewer Questions Correctly (Cumulative Frequency)
0	1	1
1	1	2
2	2	4
3	6	10
4	5	15

17.

% Who Answered This Many or Fewer Questions Correctly (Cumulative %)
1/15 = 6.7%
2/15 = 13.3%
4/15 = 26.7%
10/15 = 66.7%
15/15 = 100%

19. A scatterplot

21. A histogram better illustrates the continuum of time from one month to the next with an order involved.

23. The winery

25.

	New Cases	Deaths	Population	Mortality Rate
Men	5	2	25,000	**0.008%**
Women	3	1	25,000	**0.004%**
White	7	3	40,000	**0.0075%**
African American	1	0	10,000	**0**

DESCRIPTIVE STATISTICS, PROBABILITY, AND MEASURES OF CENTRAL TENDENCY

WHAT DOES THE DATA TELL ME?

OBJECTIVES

By the end of this chapter students will be able to:

- Compare and contrast descriptive statistics and inferential statistics.

- Define, distinguish between, and interpret the mean, median, mode, and standard deviation.

- Identify unimodal, bimodal, and multimodal distributions.

- Determine which measure of central tendency is appropriate in a given data set.

- Calculate and interpret a standard deviation and range for a given data set.

- Explain descriptive results from a given data set using an SPSS (Statistical Package for the Social Sciences) printout.

- Define probability and explain the range of possible probabilities.

- Compare and contrast frequency and probability distributions.

- Contrast positive and negative distribution skews and describe where the outliers are present.

KEY TERMS

Bimodal
Having two values or categories that have the highest occurrence and that are equal frequencies.

Central tendency
An indicator of the center of the data.

Frequency distribution
Lists all the possible outcomes of an experiment and tallies the number of times each outcome occurs.

Mean
The sum of the values divided by the total number of observations. It is the most commonly known measure of central tendency but requires interval or ratio data.

Median
For ordinal, interval, and ratio data, the value in the middle when you line up all the measured values in order from least to most; the 50th percentile value.

Mode
The most frequently occurring value or category in the distribution. When a distribution has only one mode it is called unimodal.

Multimodal
Having more than two modes.

Normal Distribution
A probability distribution in which the mean, median, and mode are equal with a bell-shaped distribution curve.

Probability
The chance that a particular outcome will occur after an event.

Probability distribution
Shows the probability of all the possible outcomes of the variable.

Range
The difference between the maximum and minimum values in a distribution.

Sampling distribution
Plots realized frequencies of a statistic versus the range of possible values that statistic can take.

Skewed Distribution
An asymmetrical distribution of the values of the variable around the mean, making one tail longer than the other.

Standard deviation
The average distance the values in a distribution are from the center.

Z-score
A standardized measure that indicates how many standard deviations a value is from the mean value.

DESCRIPTIVE STATISTICS: PROPERTIES OF VARIABLES

Once the variables of interest in a study have been defined, nurses and statisticians usually look at a set of so-called descriptive statistics that allows them to get to know more about each variable. A variable can be described in two main ways:

- In terms of its central value or tendency
- In terms of how far away from the variable's center the observations are spread

We will start by defining central tendency.

MEASURES OF CENTRAL TENDENCY

Central tendency is an indicator of the center of the data. Defining the central tendency of a distribution more specifically, however, is not easy because the answer depends on the analysis technique used—which in turn depends on the level of measurement of the data. Let's start by reviewing the levels of measurement.

First, *nominal variables* describe categorical differences, such as gender. The only measure of central tendency for nominal data is the **mode**, which is the most frequently occurring measure in the data. For example, if your sample includes 15 men and 5 women, the mode is the 15 men. This is an example of a unimodal distribution, where there is only one mode. If a ZIP code sample includes seven people living in 14617, seven people living in 14619, and six people living in 14621, the two values 14617 and 14619 have the highest occurrence and are equal, so the sample has two modes and is called **bimodal**. Large samples may even be **multimodal**; that is, they have more than two modes.

Data that is rank ordered (ordinal, interval, or ratio) has a second measure of central tendency: a **median**. If you line up all the measured values in order from least to most, the value in the middle of the list is the median. For example, suppose a set of students has the following scores on their most recent nursing exam: 66, 74, 83, 83, 88, 94, 96, 97, 99. The median score is 88, the one right in the middle. Or suppose that the first person who takes the exam forgets to hand it in, so the number of exams is even: 74, 83, 83, 88, 94, 96, 97, 99. Then the median is actually the average of the fourth and fifth values: $(88 + 94) \div 2$, or 91%.

The mode in this data is 83. You can see that the measures of central tendency do not always produce the same results. This is the main reason why defining central tendency is difficult.

Perhaps the most commonly known measure of central tendency is the **mean**, which is the sum of the values divided by the total number of observations. For example, if you add up all the original test scores and divide by the total number who took the test, you find that the mean of the original test scores is 86.67: $(66 + 74 + 83 + 83 + 88 + 94 + 96 + 97 + 99) \div 9$. Again, the mean is not the same as the median or the mode. Each is a different measure of central tendency. They may even be the same number (as in a normal distribution, which we talk about later in this chapter), but they do not have to be and they all have different definitions. The mean can be calculated only if the available data is at the interval or ratio level. You cannot calculate a mean on ordinal or nominal data. Think about it: What is the "average" gender? That doesn't make sense. Nominal or ordinal data does not lend itself to the calculation of averages. However, even with interval- or ratio-level data, you may decide to use the median instead of the mean for your measure of central tendency. This is frequently considered the better option.

Why is the median considered a better statistic to use than the mean? Students in any course should be *very* interested in the answer. Let's say the following scores are recorded on a final exam:

32, 35, 38, 40, 41, 41, 42, 43, 44, 45, 46, 47, 48, 99, 100, 100

Clearly, the class, overall, did not do very well on this exam. In fact, of the 16 people who took the exam, only 3 passed, scoring significantly higher than the rest of the class. These three scores are outliers (observations that are significantly different from the rest of the sample) and may distort the mean while leaving the median relatively unaltered. Let's take a look.

- The mean of the data is 52.6
- The median of the data is 43.5.

You can see that the 43.5 is a much better estimate of the central tendency, and in fact the mean is so high only because of the three top scores, which are very different from the rest of the data. If you scored a 48 on this test, you did fairly well in comparison to your classmates, scoring higher than 75% of them. However, what if your professor decided to look just at the mean? She might tell you that you didn't even beat the average grade for the class, even though only three people actually outscored you.

RANGE AND SAMPLE STANDARD DEVIATION

Variables can vary from their center or central tendency, and the variation can be explained by two terms.

- First, the **range** is the difference between the maximum value and minimum value of a variable. For example, in a sample there might be five subjects ages 10, 14, 20, 55, and 95. The age range of the sample is 85 years (95 years minus 10 years), or it can also be reported as 10 to 95 years.
- The **standard deviation** is the average distance of the values from the variable's mean. When the standard deviation is large, the spread among the values in the data set is large. When the deviation is

small, most of the scores are very close to the average score.

You may find that, although the average heart rate is the same on a postpartum unit as on a cardiac intensive care unit, the ranges and standard deviations in the heart rates are substantially different (see **Figure 3-1**).

Standard deviation is harder to calculate than range, but not that hard. Suppose you collect heart rates for the patients who are day 1 postdelivery on your postpartum unit and find that the mean heart rate is $(45 + 60 + 75 + 90) \div 4 = 67.5$ (see **Figure 3-2**). The formula for the standard deviation (SD) is shown in **Figure 3-3**. In a less "mathematical" version, it might look like this:

$$SD = \sqrt{\frac{(\text{first value} - \text{mean})^2 + (\text{second value} - \text{mean})^2 + \ldots + (n\text{th-mean})^2}{\text{number of values} - 1}}$$

In our example, then, the standard deviation is the square root of:

$$\frac{(45 - 67.5)^2 + (60 - 67.5)^2 + (75 - 67.5)^2 + (90 - 67.5)^2}{4 - 1}$$

FIGURE 3-1   **Heart Rate.**

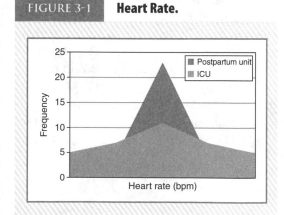

This equals:

$$\frac{(-22.5)(-22.5)+(-7.5)(-7.5)+(7.5)(7.5)+(22.5)(22.5)}{3}$$

or:

$$\frac{506.25+56.25+56.25+506.25}{3}$$

This comes down to what is actually called the sample variance:

$$\frac{1125}{3} = 375$$

Then you need to take the square root of 375: 19.36. So the standard deviation in the postpartum sample is 19.36.

FIGURE 3-2	**Frequency Table for Heart Rates Day 1 Postpartum.**

Heart Rate	Frequency
45	1
60	1
75	1
90	1

FIGURE 3-3	**Calculating the Sample Standard Deviation.**

$$SD = \sqrt{\frac{(x_1 - \mu)^2 + (x_2 - \mu)^2 + K(x_n - \mu)^2}{n-1}}$$

where
x = values in the distribution
μ = mean

FROM THE STATISTICIAN *Brendan Heavey*

Why Is There an $n - 1$ in the Denominator of Sample Variance?

Wouldn't it be a whole lot easier to remember sample variance if the denominator didn't contain an $n - 1$? The answer is yes, remembering the formula would be a heck of a lot easier if we could just scrap the $n - 1$ and throw an n into the denominator. In fact, as the sample size of our data set increases, the $n - 1$ becomes more and more negligible. However, in small samples we can see that the sample mean is a lot closer to each sample value than the population mean.

Think about it: Although the sample mean is a decent descriptor of the middle of our sample, the population mean doesn't even have to be within the range of our sample! Let's think about an example. If you were interested in estimating the average heart rate of a human being in normal sinus rhythm you might sample from 10 different healthy volunteers. Each volunteer would have small differences in individual heart rate depending on what time of day you took their pulses, how much they had been moving in the moments leading up to your measurement, their body mass index (BMI), and so on. Let's say you chose to

(continues)

FROM THE STATISTICIAN   *Brendan Heavey*

test each person's heart rate five different times, and took an average of those measurements to report on; your results might look like this:

Heart Rates Measured at Five Different Times

	Person 1	Person 2	Person 3	Person 4	Person 5
	65	65	51	69	79
	62	67	58	72	72
	60	58	55	73	75
	58	62	53	70	78
	61	63	59	76	77
Sample Means	Avg = 61.2	Avg = 63	Avg = 55.2	Avg = 72	Avg = 76.2
Population Mean			Overall Average = 65.52		

Take a look at how the individual pulse rates vary around their individual sample means. Notice that the overall mean is generally further away from the data points than the sample mean is. In fact, the population mean is not even in the range of Person 5's recorded values. Let's calculate the numerator of Person 5's variance using the sample mean. We get:

$$(79 - 76.2)^2 + (72 - 76.2)^2 + (75 - 76.2)^2 + (78 - 76.2)^2 + (77 - 76.2)^2 = 30.8$$

Now, let's do the same thing but substitute the population mean. We get:

$$(79 - 65.52)^2 + (72 - 65.52)^2 + (75 - 65.52)^2 + (78 - 65.52)^2 + (77 - 65.52)^2 = 60.112$$

Clearly, Person 5 contributes a lot more to the variance component of the population than he or she does to the sample. In general, there is a lot less variance around the sample mean than the population mean, so sample variance tends to underestimate the population variance. You can make up for this difference, or what the statisticians call bias, by putting an $n - 1$ in the denominator of the sample variance calculation.

Okay, now I know some of you are starting to wonder, "Why am I in this class again?" Don't get too frustrated by the equations. (If, on the other hand, you are just dying to know more about variance, please read the "From the Statistician" feature, which delves further into this topic.) The essential concept to understand is why the standard deviation is important. (*It tells you the average distance the values in your distribution fall from the mean.*)

MOVING FORWARD: INFERENTIAL STATISTICS

Once researchers are done describing the variables they are interested in, they usually like to make inferences about populations based on the measurements they have taken in their samples. This practice, called inferential statistics, involves associating probabilities with each variable studied. **Probability** is the chance that a particular outcome will occur. For example, let's say a class of 100 nursing students has 25 men and 75 women, and we want to know the probability that a randomly chosen student from this class will be female. The answer is 75/100, or 0.75, or 75%. Probabilities are important because, no matter how careful and precise researchers are, there is always some level of uncertainty. Even if the researchers believe the class is composed entirely of men, the researchers cannot say the probability is 1.0, or 100%, that a randomly chosen student will be male; they can only say that the probability approaches 100%. (Did anyone see the Disney movie *Mulan*? To make a long story short, a young

FROM THE STATISTICIAN *Brendan Heavey*

Probability and the Normal Distribution

Probability is a difficult concept to fully grasp. In fact, it has so many different facets that at times statisticians have a difficult time adequately defining it. The good news is that, at this point, you don't need an extremely in-depth understanding of it. In fact, for the purposes of this text, think of probability as long-run relative frequency. You should know what relative frequency means, but what does "long-run" mean? That is an important question, and it doesn't have a very good answer. Let's look at an example to try to explain this concept.

We are going to revisit the age-old experiment of rolling dice. **Figure 3-4** shows the results of rolling a single die 10 times and counting how many times the die shows a 3 on its face. The cumulative and relative frequencies associated with each roll are tabulated in the last two columns. This time, we're going to focus on the final column, the relative frequency. The relative frequency is the total number of times you roll a particular value (in this case, 3) out of the total number of rolls.

If you look at the relative frequency column closely, you will notice that it starts out low and then, as soon as we roll a 3, the relative frequency jumps up to 0.5. In fact, if we continued this experiment for a long time, the jumping would continue forever—each time you roll another 3 and increase the numerator. However, each jump would be smaller than the last (because each roll also increases the denominator).

Just for fun, we did this very thing and plotted the relative frequency over 1,000 rolls in **Figure 3-5**. Notice that, after a while, the relative frequency of rolling a 3 settles down to around 0.16, or 1/6. In the beginning, the relative frequency jumps up and down, but after about 100 rolls, we can clearly see the trend settling. We would fully expect this going forward because the die has six sides, and if we rolled the die a million times, we would expect somewhere around 1/6 of them to turn up a 3. In this experiment, because we can see the main pattern developed after 100 rolls, we would define "long run" as 100 rolls, but keep in mind that the definition can change between experiments.

FIGURE 3-4   **Frequency Table for Rolling a 3 When Rolling a Six-Sided Die.**

Roll	Result	Cumulative Frequency of 3	Relative Frequency of 3
1	1	0	0
2	3	1	$\frac{1}{2} = 0.5$
3	2	1	$\frac{1}{3} = 0.33$
4	5	1	$\frac{1}{4} = 0.25$
5	6	1	$\frac{1}{5} = 0.2$
6	2	1	$\frac{1}{6} = 0.16$
7	3	2	$\frac{1}{7} = 0.29$
8	4	2	$\frac{2}{8} = 0.25$
9	4	2	$\frac{2}{9} = 0.22$
10	6	2	$\frac{2}{10} = 0.2$

FIGURE 3-5   **Graph of the Relative Frequency of Rolling a 3.**

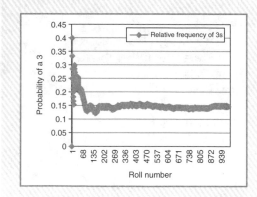

Chinese woman joins the imperial army disguised as a man. If one were to randomly select an infantry soldier from this "all-male" group, the probability that you would select a man approaches 100%, but there is always room for some error, such as if one were to randomly select Mulan in disguise. But I digress….) Conversely, the researchers cannot say that the probability of randomly selecting a female from what they believe is an all-male class is 0.0, or 0%. They can only say the probability approaches 0. Probability theory is a science in and of itself, so here we will cover it in a nutshell in the next "From the Statistician."

FREQUENCY DISTRIBUTIONS VERSUS PROBABILITY DISTRIBUTIONS

You may remember that a **frequency distribution** simply lists all the possible outcomes of an experiment and tallies the number of times each outcome occurs. These tallies are then graphed to make them easier to visualize and comprehend. A **probability distribution** graphs the probability of all the possible outcomes of the variable instead of their frequency. Although they both look a lot alike, they represent two very distinct concepts.

Let's look more in depth at the difference between a frequency distribution and a probability distribution. The frequency distribution for the experiment of rolling a die 1,000 times is shown in **Figure 3-6** and compared against the probability distribution of rolling a die indefinitely. As you can

see, the frequency distribution has notches and changes depending on what a sample looks like. The probability distribution is uniform and never changes. The relationship between relative frequency and probability closely resembles the relationship between a sample and a population. The difference boils down to a basic difference between the short run (100 tosses of the die) and the long run (1,000, 10,000, 100,000 tosses), and defining the long run is slightly subjective.

"That's great," you might say, "But I'm a nurse! I'm never going to need to roll dice

FIGURE 3-6   **Frequency versus Probability Distribution.**

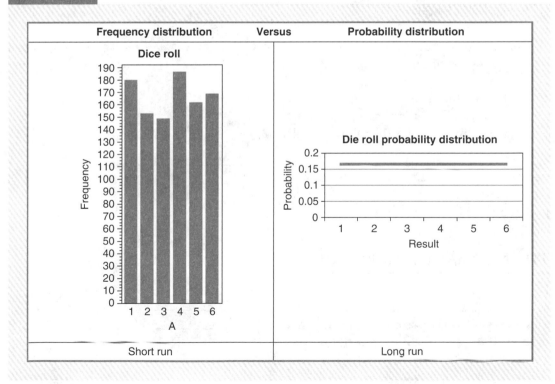

and come up with associated probabilities unless I meet a poor statistician sitting at a bar all alone somewhere!" Nevertheless, as it turns out, rolling a die is just a very straightforward example of an experiment. Let's consider a couple of basic experiments and see how they might relate to your life and profession. For instance, we can now easily answer the following:

- What is the long-run relative frequency (or probability) of a fair coin turning up heads?
- What is the long-run relative frequency (or probability) of a fair die rolling a 6?

Now, let's look at answering some questions we're more interested in:

- What is the probability that I will die of cardiovascular disease?
- What is the probability that one of my patients will be discharged before I come back to the hospital to work my next shift?
- What is the probability that a new drug will kill a cancerous tumor in my patient's liver without killing my patient?

Answering these questions with any degree of accuracy requires a lot of study, a lot of repeated samples, and determining probability—as you just did.

THE NORMAL DISTRIBUTION

Many variables of interest to us have a probability distribution that closely resembles a very famous distribution: the **normal distribution**, a probability distribution in which the mean, median, and mode are equal (see **Figure 3-7**). In fact, one of the most common assumptions in basic research is that the variables have probability distributions that can be estimated with the normal distribution. The normal distribution is what all of us have heard of as the "bell curve." Yes, this is how grades are "curved" when no one does well on a test. Many people believe that, given a well-constructed exam administered to a large enough sample, we should expect a grade distribution that can be estimated with the normal distribution.

Because in the normal distribution the mean, median, and mode are the same, you know two things about a variable that is normally distributed (see **Figure 3-7**):

- Sixty-eight percent of its values fall within one standard deviation of the mean.
- Ninety-five percent of its values fall within two standard deviations of the mean.

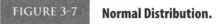

FIGURE 3-7   **Normal Distribution.**

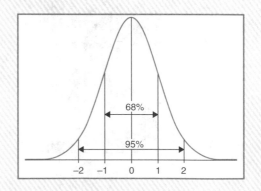

FROM THE STATISTICIAN *Brendan Heavey*

What is a Normal Distribution?

For most researchers, the normal distribution is the most important distribution in all of statistics. Two very important facts about the normal distribution make it so important:

1. If you take the mean from lots and lots of samples of a population, the distribution of the sample means (the sampling distribution of the mean) becomes normal in the long run. **Sampling distributions** plot *actual* frequencies of a statistic versus the range of *possible* values that statistic can take.
2. As you add more and more random variables together, their overall distribution approaches the normal distribution.

In **Figure 3-8**, check out how the plot of the normal distribution looks as you adjust its mean. As the mean (μ) of the distribution increases in these graphs, the curve shifts to the right; as it decreases, the curve shifts to the left. This shift is why we call the mean a location parameter.

In **Figure 3-9**, see what happens when we change the variance. If we were to change only the variance (σ) in our formula, we would see a change in scale. As we decrease the variance, the graph gets taller and skinnier, and as we increase it, the graph gets shorter and fatter. That is why variance is called a scale variable.

Here are some more important things we know about the normal distribution:

- Sixty-eight percent of the area under the curve falls within 1 standard deviation of the mean.
- Ninety-five percent of the area under the curve falls within 2 standard deviations of the mean.
- Increasing the mean makes the curve shift to the right.
- Decreasing the mean makes the curve shift to the left.
- Decreasing the variance makes the graph look taller and skinnier.
- Increasing the variance makes it look shorter and fatter.

An important thing we can do with any normal variable is transform its distribution into a *standard* normal distribution. This forces all the area under the curve to fall under the normal curve with a mean of 0 and a standard deviation of 1. We do this with the transformation formula shown in **Figure 3-10**. If Y is a normally distributed variable, this equation will produce Z, which is a standard normal variable. Standard normal variables are great because we know a lot about their probabilities. For instance, 5% of the probability is found beyond $Z = 1.96$.

SKEWED DISTRIBUTIONS

Of course, not all samples are normally distributed. For example, some samples are skewed; they have an asymmetrical distribution of the values of the variable around the mean so that one tail is longer than the other (see **Figure 3-11**). Skewing is usually due to a

| FIGURE 3-8 | **Normal Distribution: Changing the Mean.** |

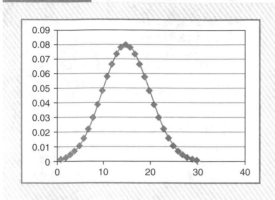 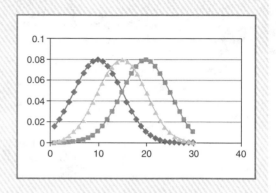

| FIGURE 3-9 | **Normal Distribution: Changing the Variance.** |

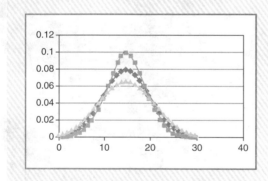

| FIGURE 3-10 | **Formula for Creating a Standard Normal Variable with Population Data.** |

$$Z = \frac{Y - \mu}{\sigma} \sim N(0,1)$$

significant number of outliers. When the outliers are on the right, the skew is positive; if most of the outliers are on the left, the skew is negative. In skewed distributions, the mean, median, and mode are not equal. Remember the test where you got a 48 but only three people scored higher? That is an example of a positive skew produced by outliers.

Another interesting thing we can do when we have a normal distribution is to calculate a test statistic called a **Z-score**. Z-scores are a standardized measure that tells you how many standard deviations the observation is from the mean. If a value in a data set is above the mean or average it will have a positive Z-score. If it is below the mean or average it will have a negative Z-score. The larger the absolute value of the Z-score, the further the value is from the average or mean value in the data set. For example, a nurse educator gives a pretest to a group of newly diagnosed diabetics before teaching about insulin injection techniques. The test score is normally distributed with an average score of 70% and a standard deviation of four points. The Z-score for a test value of 70% is 0, and a Z-score of 1.0 corresponds to

Skewed Distributions.

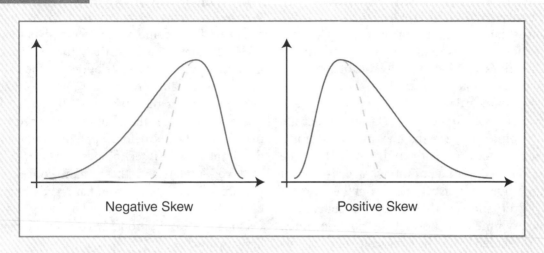

Negative Skew   Positive Skew

a test score of 74%. A Z-score of 2.0 lies 2.0 standard deviations above the mean and, in this example, corresponds to a test score of 78%; in contrast, a Z-score of −0.5 lies 0.5 standard deviations below the mean, or in this example a test score of 68%. The formula for calculating Z-scores in a population is shown in Figure 3-10 and is just the observed value minus the mean which is then divided by the standard deviation.

Z-scores can be helpful because we know the associated probability (such as 95%) of the values fall between two standard deviations or Z-scores of approximately −2 to +2. Z-scores are also standardized so we can use them to compare different values from different data sets. For example, an orthopedic rehabilitation patient with a functional mobility test score of 12 and a corresponding Z-score value of 1 and a range of motion score of 17 with a corresponding Z-score of −0.5 means the patient is doing better than the population average in functional mobility but worse than

the population average in range of motion. The absolute value of the test score does not tell us the relationship this score may have to the usual or expected outcomes in the field, but a Z-score may give us that information.

SUMMARY

Congratulate yourself for making it through this chapter! Let's restate some main points from this very detailed chapter.

When you have nominal-level data, the only measure of central tendency you can use is the mode. The mode is the most frequently occurring measure in a distribution. A bimodal distribution has two values with the highest number of frequencies an equal number of times; this gives you two modes. Taking that one step further, a multimodal distribution has more than two modes.

The median can be used with ordinal, interval, or ratio data and is found by lining up the measured values in order from least to greatest and locating the value in the middle. For interval- or ratio-level data, you can also calculate a mean or average. The mean is the most commonly known measure of central tendency and is found by taking the sum of the values and dividing it by the total number of observations.

With regard to the dispersion of your data, two terms are important: (1) the range, or the difference between the maximum and minimum values in the distribution, and (2) the standard deviation, or the average distance of the values in a distribution from the center.

Everyone's favorite concept in statistics is the symmetrical normal distribution, often represented by the bell curve. If your data fits into this type of distribution, it simplifies your analysis immensely. It also lets you calculate Z-scores, which are standardized scores that can be useful in comparing different data sets.

Some samples are skewed; that is, they have an asymmetrical distribution of the values of the variable around the mean so that one tail is larger than the other. If you have this type of sample distribution, you need to make adjustments before applying some of the simpler analysis techniques.

If you understand these main concepts, you are on the right track and are ready to go on to the next chapter—or take a long nap. Personally, I would probably vote for the nap first anyhow!

CHAPTER 3 REVIEW QUESTIONS

Questions 1–5: Your results are 2, 14, 6, 8, 10, 4, 12, 8.

1. What is the mean?

2. What is the median?

3. What is the mode?

4. Calculate the standard deviation.

5. If the sample is normally distributed, 68% of the responses are within what range?

6. If a study reports that you have a normally distributed sample with a mean age of 17.3 years, what is the median?

Questions 7–12: A study polls 40 new mothers who attempt to nurse their infants from birth to 6 weeks. Twenty-seven mothers report nursing with minimal pain and frustration, 10 mothers report nursing with moderate pain and frustration, and 3 mothers report discontinuing nursing due to high levels of pain and frustration.

7. What is the mode for nursing pain and frustration?

8. What is the median for nursing pain and frustration?

9. What percentage of mothers continued to nurse for the full 6 weeks with minimal pain and frustration?

10. What percentage of mothers reported less than or equal to moderate pain and frustration?

11. What level of measurement is the nursing pain and frustration?

12. How could you increase the level of measurement?

Questions 13–18: You read a study involving a new screen for rheumatoid arthritis, and the report indicates that those with the disease had the antibody levels shown in **Figure 3-12**.

FIGURE 3-12 **Frequency Table for Rheumatoid Arthritis Screen.**

Antibody Level	Frequency	Cumulative Frequency
20	3	—
30	5	—
43	3	—
48	7	—

13. Complete the cumulative frequency column.
14. How many subjects had their antibody levels reported?

15. What antibody level was the mode?

16. What antibody level was the median?

17. What antibody level was the mean?

18. Is this sample normally distributed?

Questions 19–21: Final exam grades are normally distributed with a mean of 81. The standard deviation is 3.

19. What range includes 68% of the sample?

20. What range includes 95% of the sample?

21. What is the median grade?

Questions 22–26: A researcher is measuring how many times a minute a person coughs when exposed to cigarette smoke. The results from the study are normally distributed, and they include a mean of 4 and a standard deviation of 2.

22. What level of measurement is this?

23. What is an appropriate measure of central tendency?

24. Where do 68% of the sample responses fall?

25. If instead the results show a mean of 4 and a standard deviation of 1 but they remain normally distributed, what would this change do to the curve?

26. The follow-up cohort study reports a mean of 5 and a standard deviation of 1. What would this change do to the curve?

Questions 27–31: A sample of eight orthopedic patients on your unit includes two patients on intravenous anticoagulants, four patients on oral anticoagulants, and two patients on subcutaneous anticoagulants.

27. Based on this sample, calculate the probability that orthopedic patients are given IV anticoagulants.

28. Calculate the probability that orthopedic patients are given oral anticoagulants.

29. Calculate the probability that orthopedic patients are given subcutaneous anticoagulants.

30. Based on this sample, what is the probability that an orthopedic patient will be given some form of anticoagulant?

31. Hip replacement patients have the same probability of being on oral anticoagulants as the orthopedic patients in your previous study, and you have four in your daily assignment. Calculate the number of patients with hip replacements who you would anticipate would need oral anticoagulants.

Questions 32–40: A researcher is comparing patients with high medication compliance versus those with low medication compliance in an outpatient psychiatric day program utilizing the Hamilton Anxiety Rating Scale (HAM-A), which has 14 items scored on a scale of 1–4. A higher score on the HAM-A indicates higher levels of anxiety. After collecting the data, she determines the scores obtained in both groups are normally distributed. In the low compliance group, the mean score is 24 and the standard deviation is 2. In the high compliance group, the mean score is 16 and the standard deviation is 1.5.

32. What level of measurement are the instrument items?

33. What is the median score in the low compliance group?

34. A patient in the low compliance group scores 26. Is this patient more or less anxious than average in this group?

35. Another patient in the low compliance group has a score with a corresponding Z-score of -1.5. What was his actual HAM-A score? Was he more or less anxious than the average patient in this group?

36. The researcher knows that with these results, 68% of her subjects in the low compliance group scored in what range on the HAM-A?

37. A patient in the high compliance group has a score with a corresponding Z-score of 2. What was her actual HAM-A score? Is she more or less anxious than the average patient in this group?

38. If the researcher graphs the frequency distributions for the scores in each of the two groups, which group will have a flatter bell curve? Why?

39. If instead of finding a normal distribution in the low compliance group the researcher discovers there are three individuals with scores that are substantially higher than the rest of the group, what type of skew would these outliers cause?

40. If the distribution is skewed, what do you know about the mean, median, and mode?

ANSWERS TO CHAPTER 3 REVIEW QUESTIONS

1. 8

3. 8

5. Between 4 and 12

7. Minimal

9. 67.5%

11. Ordinal

13. 3, 8, 11, 18

15. Mode = 48

17. Mean = 37.5

19. 78–84

21. 81

23. Any

25. Make it taller and skinnier

27. $\frac{2}{8} = \frac{1}{4} = 25\%$

29. $\frac{2}{8} = \frac{1}{4} = 25\%$

31. 2

33. 24

35. 21, less anxious

37. 19, more anxious

39. Positive skew

EVALUATING YOUR MEASUREMENT TOOL

IS YOUR INSTRUMENT GOOD, BAD, OR UGLY?

OBJECTIVES

By the end of the chapter students will be able to:

- Discuss factors that impact the feasibility of a study.
- Define validity and why it is essential in research.
- Identify various methods for establishing validity, and give an example of each.
- Define reliability and relate why it is important in research.
- Describe the main components of reliability.
- Detect when inter-rater reliability needs to be assessed and develop a plan for doing so.
- Formulate a 2 × 2 table, and calculate the sensitivity and specificity of a screening test from a given data set.

- Distinguish between sensitivity and specificity, and identify when each is important.
- Calculate the positive and negative predictive values of a screening test.
- Calculate the prevalence of an illness and describe how the positive and negative predictive values of the screening test are affected by the prevalence of the illness among the test population.
- Critique a screening test utilizing a given data set.
- Prepare an argument for why or why not a particular screen should be utilized based on current research.

KEY TERMS

Content validity
When the instrument used is designed to accurately measure the concepts under study.

Convergent validity
When the results obtained are similar to the results obtained with another previously validated test that measures the same thing.

Correlation Coefficient
A test value used to determine how closely one measurement is related to a second measurement.

Divergent validity
When the measurement of the opposite variable of a previously validated measurement yields the opposite result.

Efficiency (EFF)
Measures the probability of agreement between the screening test and the actual clinical diagnosis.

Equivalence
How well multiple forms or multiple users of an instrument produce the same results.

Feasible
Possible from a practical standpoint.

Homogeneity
The extent to which items on a multi-item instrument are consistent with one another.

Internal consistency reliability
Homogeneity of the measurement instrument.

Inter-rater reliability
When you compare the measurements obtained by two different data collectors to make sure they are similar.

Negative predictive value
If the subject tests negative for a disease, the probability that the subject really doesn't have the disease.

Positive predictive value (PPV)
If a subject tests positive for a disease, the probability that the subject actually has the disease and that the result isn't a false positive.

Predictive validity
When the instrument used accurately suggests future outcomes or behaviors.

Prevalence
The amount of illness present in the population divided by the total population.

Reliability
The consistency or repeatability of the measurement.

Sensitivity
If the patient has a disease, the probability of a positive test result for the disease (the probability of a true positive).

Specificity
The probability that a well subject will have a negative screen (no disease) (the probability of a true negative).

Stability
The consistent or enduring quality of the measure.

Valid
Accurate.

FEASIBILITY

Before selecting any type of research instrument you should always assess how **feasible** or practical the tool is. If, for example, you want to use computer-assisted interviewing techniques to survey adolescents about sexual behavior, but your grant is for $1,000 and each device costs $1,200, it is probably not a practical plan. A study that involves asking patients with dementia to complete a 24-hour recall of food consumption also lacks feasibility. A wise nurse will consider the practical aspects of the study's measurement tool such as the cost, time, training, and limitations of the study sample (physical, cultural, educational, psychosocial, etc.) before beginning the analysis of the validity and reliability of the instruments themselves.

VALIDITY

After you determine that your instrument is feasible for use in your study, you can then proceed to assess the validity and reliability of your tool. The information you gather is helpful only if your measurement and collection methods are accurate, or **valid**. You can ensure that an instrument has validity in several ways:

- *Determine relevant variables by conducting a thorough literature search.* When you began your research, you did a literature search to determine what information, if any, was already available about the relationship between family visits and the length of recovery time needed after a hip replacement.
- *Include the variables in a measurement instrument.* In your literature search, you identified some of the major variables to consider in your study, such as the support level of family members, the age

of the patient, whether the patient lives alone, whether this was the patient's first surgery, and other factors.

- *Have your instrument reviewed by experts for feedback.* When you designed the survey for your study, you included these variables and then had your nurse manager, two nursing researchers, and your fellowship advisor (all experts) review your survey.

These steps are all part of ensuring **content validity**.

You can also show validity in your survey by comparing your results with those of a previously validated survey that measures the same thing. This type of comparison is called **convergent validity**. For example, if you find a correlation of 0.4 or higher, that finding strengthens the validity of both instruments, yours and the previous one (Grove, 2007). In turn, if your survey is later found to be able to predict the length of stay for those admitted in the future, that finding will strengthen the validity of your instrument and your study would have **predictive validity** as well.

Some instruments are considered valid because they measure the opposite variable of a previously validated measurement and find the opposite result. For instance, suppose a group of people with elevated serum cholesterol levels also scored low on a survey you designed to measure intake of fruits and vegetables. This result is an example of **divergent validity** in your instrument. The group with high cholesterol also had a poor diet. If the negative correlation is greater than or equal to −0.4, the divergent validity of both measures is strengthened (Grove, 2007).

Another way to show validity with opposite results is if your instrument detects a difference in groups already known to have a difference.

This is also referred to as construct validity testing using known groups. For example, you are testing a new instrument to examine labor outcomes in women who have already had a baby versus those experiencing their first labor. The instrument measures length of labor, which has already been shown to be shorter for women who have had a baby. You find that those who have had a baby have a length of labor that is on average 2 hours shorter than those who have not. This finding supports the validity of your new measurement tool because it detected a difference that was known to exist.

RELIABILITY

Reliability means that your measurement tool is consistent or repeatable. When you measure your variable of interest, do you get the same results every time? Reliability is different from accuracy or validity. Suppose, for example, that you are measuring the weight of the study participants, but your scale is not calibrated correctly; it is off by 20 pounds. You get the same measure every time the patient steps on the scale; that is, the measurement is repeatable and reliable. However, in this case it is not accurate or valid. A measure can be reliable and not valid, but it can't be valid and not reliable. Think of it this way: For an instrument to be accurate (valid), it must be accurate and reliable.

Three main factors relate to reliability: stability, homogeneity, and equivalence. **Stability** is the consistent or enduring quality of the measure. A stable measure:

- Should not change over time.
- When administered repeatedly, should have a high correlation coefficient. (The correlation coefficient measures how closely one measurement is related to a second measurement. For example, if

you measure the temperature of a healthy individual six times in an hour, the readings should be approximately the same and have a high correlation coefficient. Of course, that patient may be really sick of having you around, but I am sure your excitement at discovering that you have a stable measure will make it all worthwhile!)

You need to evaluate the stability of your measurement instrument at the beginning of the study and throughout it. For example, if your thermometer breaks, the instrument that was once stable is no longer available. Your ongoing results are no longer reliable, and you need to have a protocol to figure out quickly how to reestablish stability.

The second quality of a reliable measure, **homogeneity**, is the extent to which items on a multi-item instrument are consistent with one another. For example, your survey may ask several questions designed to measure the level of family support. The questions may be repeated but worded differently to see whether the individuals completing the survey respond in the same way. One question may ask, "What level of family support do you feel on most days?", and the choices may be high, medium, and low. Later in the survey you may ask the individual to indicate on a scale of 1 to 10 the degree of family support felt on an average day. If the instrument has homogeneity, those who answered that they had, say, a medium level of family support on most days should also be somewhere around the middle of the 1–10 scale. If so, then your instrument is said to have **internal consistency reliability**.

Internal consistency reliability is useful for instruments that measure a single concept, such as family support, and is frequently assessed using Cronbach's alpha. Cronbach's alpha ranges from 0 (no reliability in the instrument scale) to 1 (perfect reliability in the instrument scale), so a higher value indicates better internal consistency reliability. You may hear more about this test in future statistics or research classes, but right now you just need to know that it can be used to establish homogeneity or internal consistency reliability (Nieswiadomy, 2008).

The third factor relating to reliability is **equivalence**. Equivalence is how well multiple forms of an instrument or multiple users of an instrument produce/obtain the same results. Measurement variation is a reflection of more than the reliability of the tool itself; it may also reflect the variability of different forms of the tool or variability due to different researchers administering the same tool. For example, if you want to observe the color of scrubs worn by 60 nurses at lunchtime on a particular day, you might need help in gathering that much data in such a short period of time. You might ask two research assistants to observe the nurses. When you have more than one individual collecting data, you should determine the **inter-rater reliability**. One way to do this is to have all three individuals who are collecting data observe the first five nurses together and then classify the data individually. For example:

- You say the first five nurses are wearing blue, green, green, orange, and pink scrubs.
- The second research assistant reports that the first five nurses are wearing teal, lime, lime, tangerine, and rose scrubs.
- The third reports that the first five nurses are wearing blue, green, green, orange, and pink scrubs.

In this example, the inter-rater reliability between you and the third data collector is 100%, whereas it is 0% between you and the second collector. You have clearly identified a problem with the instrument's inter-rater reliability.

One way to increase reliability is to create color categories for data collection; for example, blue, green, orange, yellow, and other. In this case:

- You report the first five nurses are wearing blue, green, green, orange, and other.
- The second data collector reports the nurses are wearing blue, green, green, other, and other.
- The third data collector matches your selections again.

Clearly you have improved the inter-rater reliability, but some variability is left due to the collectors' differences in interpretation of colors. With this information, you may decide that the help of the second data collector isn't worth the loss in inter-rater reliability. You might run the study with only two data collectors, or you may decide to sit down, define specific colors with the second data collector, and then reexamine the inter-rater reliability. In all such cases, you must consider this concern whenever the study requires more than one data collector.

The readability of an instrument can also affect both the validity and the reliability of the tool. If your study participants cannot understand the words in your survey tool, there is a very good chance they will not complete it accurately or consistently and that would ruin all your hard work. A good researcher assesses the readability of his or her instrument before or during the pilot stage of a study.

One last point to remember is that the validity and reliability of an instrument are not inherent attributes of the instrument but are characteristics of the use of the instrument with a particular group of respondents at a particular time. For example, an instrument that has been shown to be valid and reliable when used with an urban elderly population may not be valid and reliable when used with a rural adolescent population. For this reason, the validity and reliability of an instrument should be reassessed whenever that instrument is used in a new situation.

SCREENING TESTS

Different but related terms are utilized when a screening test is selected. The accuracy of a screening test is determined by its ability to identify subjects who have the disease and subjects who do not. However, accuracy does not mean that all subjects who have a positive screen have the disease and that all subjects who have a negative screen do not.

The four possible outcomes from any screening test are best illustrated in a standard 2 × 2 table, also called a contingency table (see **Figure 4-1**).

- If a subject actually has the disease and the screen is positive, the result is a true positive and belongs in the first box (*A*).
- If the subject does not have the disease and the screen is positive, it is a false positive and belongs in the second box (*B*).
- If the subject has the disease and tests negative, it is a false negative result and belongs in the third box (*C*).
- If the subject does not have the disease and the screen is negative, it is a true negative and belongs in the fourth box (*D*).

SENSITIVITY

When evaluating a screening test, one of the things nurses like to know is, if the patient has the disease, what is the probability that he or she will test positive for the disease. This is known as the **sensitivity** of the test and can be calculated by the equation in **Figure 4-2**. Intuitively, this equation should make sense. Take the number of subjects who are sick and test positive, and divide this number by the total number of subjects who are ill. It is a matter of percentages: the number who are really sick and who test positive divided by the total number of people who really are sick. If a screen is sensitive, it is very good at identifying people who are actually sick, and it has a low percentage of false negatives. Sensitivity is particularly important when a disease is fatal or contagious or when early treatment helps.

FIGURE 4-2 **Formula to Calculate the Sensitivity of a Screen.**

$$\text{Sensitivity} = \frac{A \ (\text{True positives})}{A + C \ (\text{All who have the disease})}$$

FIGURE 4-1 **A 2 × 2 Table.**

	Disease Present	Disease Not Present
Test Positive	True positive (*A*)	False positive (*B*)
Test Negative	False negative (*C*)	True negative (*D*)

SPECIFICITY

Another piece of information that helps evaluate a screening tool is the **specificity**, or the probability that a well subject will have a negative screen (no disease). Using the same 2 × 2 table, **specificity** can be calculated with the equation in **Figure 4-3**. Similar to the previous equation, this equation takes the number of people who are not ill and who have a negative screening test and divides this number by the total number of people who are not ill. When a screen is highly specific, it is very good at identifying subjects who are not ill and has a low percentage of false positives.

Sensitivity and specificity tend to work in a converse balance with each other, and sometimes a loss in one is traded for an improvement in another. For example, suppose you are a nurse working on an infectious disease outbreak in a mobile military unit overseas. Your ability to find these patients again is very limited, so you want to be as certain as possible that those you screen negative

| FIGURE 4-3 | **Formula to Calculate the Specificity of a Screen.** |

$$\text{Specificity} = \frac{\text{True negatives } (D)}{\text{All those who do not have the disease } (B + D)}$$

and who leave the mobile facility are not really carrying the disease for which you are screening. Because of this you select a highly specific test that is very good at identifying those who do not have the disease for which you are screening. It rarely says a healthy person is sick. When a highly specific test is negative you know the chances are very good that the person is actually healthy and can leave the facility without a concern that they could spread the disease for which you are screening. You can then hold or contain those who do test positive for further testing and evaluation.

FROM THE STATISTICIAN *Brendan Heavey*

Sensitivity and Specificity

Let's review some concepts in this chapter in the context of testing a large group of individuals for tuberculosis. For instance, when you entered nursing school, you were probably subjected to tests to determine whether you carried tuberculosis. The first step in the testing process is a Purified Protein Derivative (PPD), which shows whether a person has antibodies to the bacterium that causes tuberculosis. A person who responds to this test may be asked to undergo any number of tests, including:

- Chest x-ray
- Biopsy
- Urine culture

(continues)

FROM THE STATISTICIAN *Brendan Heavey*

- Cerebrospinal fluid sample
- Computed tomography (CT) scan
- Magnetic resonance imaging (MRI) scan

Each of these tests has a number of different characteristics. They can all be used in the diagnosis of tuberculosis infection, but which test is best? This question turns out to be very challenging, and the answer depends on the definition of "best." Further, each person's definition of best can be different and can change depending on that individual's perception of reality. For instance, each test costs a different amount to administer, so is the cheapest test the best? (If you thought you had tuberculosis, cost would probably not be your criterion for best.) Each test also ranges in its degree of invasiveness. Would you want to be subjected to a cerebrospinal fluid sample (which is very painful) if you didn't think you had the disease and just wanted to get into nursing school?

Each of these tests has a different sensitivity and specificity. A very important trait of each test that you should be interested in knowing is how often a person with tuberculosis is actually diagnosed correctly. A second trait of interest is how often a person without tuberculosis is correctly diagnosed. In general, a high sensitivity/lower specificity test is administered first to determine a large set of people who *may* have the disease. Sensitive tests are very good at identifying those who have a disease. Then additional costs and tests are incurred to increase specificity, or eliminate people who are actually healthy (and were false positives) before diagnosis and treatment begin.

This approach is like using a microscope. The first step is to use a low-resolution lens to find the area of a slide that you are interested in. Then you increase the resolution to look more closely at the object of interest. A test with high sensitivity/low specificity is like a low-resolution lens to identify those who may have the disease. As you increase specificity, you narrow down the population of interest and eliminate those who were falsely testing positive. An example of this practice is included in Doering et al. (2007).

POSITIVE PREDICTIVE VALUE OF A SCREEN

Another important concept to understand about any screening test is **positive predictive value (PPV)**. PPV tells you what the probability is that a subject actually has the disease given a positive test result—that is, the probability of a true positive. Look back at the 2 × 2 table in Figure 4-1. You can calculate the PPV with the equation in **Figure 4-4**.

FIGURE 4-4 **Formula to Calculate the Positive Predictive Value of a Screen.**

$$PPV = \frac{\text{True positives } (A)}{\text{Total number who tested positive } (A + B)}$$

Unfortunately, many students find this concept confusing because it depends not just on the sensitivity and specificity of the test, but also on the **prevalence** of the illness in the population you are screening. Prevalence is the amount of illness (the number of cases) present in the population divided by the total population. If you look back at the 2 × 2 table, you can determine the prevalence quite easily. It is just the number of people who have the disease divided by the total population (see **Figure 4-5**).

If you administer a screening test with an established sensitivity and specificity in a population with a high prevalence of the disease, your screening will have a heightened positive predictive value. If the population does not have a high prevalence of the disease, PPV is decreased. Even without looking at the 2 × 2 table, this phenomenon makes intuitive sense. If you are looking for a disease that is very rare, a positive test result in that population is more likely to be a false positive than in a population where 90% of the population actually has the disease.

NEGATIVE PREDICTIVE VALUE

A related concept is the **negative predictive value (NPV)** of a test: If your subject screens negatively, NPV tells you the probability that the patient really does not have the disease. Like PPV, this measure depends on sensitivity, specificity, and the prevalence of the illness in the population where you are administering the test. Using the 2 × 2 table again, you can determine the NPV using the equation in **Figure 4-6**.

EFFICIENCY

One last concept is particularly useful in a clinical setting. **Efficiency (EFF)** is a measure of the agreement between the screening test and the actual clinical diagnosis. To determine efficiency, add all the true positives and all the true negatives and determine what proportion of your sample that is. (This is the group the test correctly identified and, therefore, the diagnosis is made correctly. That is always a good thing in nursing!) Efficiency can be calculated by using the formula in **Figure 4-7**.

FIGURE 4-6 **Formula to Calculate Negative Predictive Value (NPV) from a 2 × 2 Table.**

$$NPV = \frac{\text{True negatives } (D)}{\text{All the subjects who tested negative } (C + D)}$$

FIGURE 4-5 **Formula to Calculate Prevalence from A 2 × 2 Table.**

$$Prevalence = \frac{A + C}{A + B + C + D}$$

FIGURE 4-7 **Formula for Calculating Efficiency (EFF).**

$$EFF = \frac{A + D}{A + B + C + D} \times 100$$

SUMMARY

You have completed the chapter and are doing a great job! Let's recap the main ideas.

Validity is the accuracy of your measurement. To assess content validity, determine the relevant variables from a thorough literature search, include them in your measurement instrument, and have your instrument reviewed by experts for feedback. For convergent validity, you compare your results with those of another previously validated survey that measured the same thing. Divergent validity is the opposite: It measures the opposite variable of a previously validated measurement and finds the opposite result.

Reliability tells you whether your measurement tool is consistent or repeatable. Stability is one of the main factors that contributes to reliability and is the consistent or enduring quality of the measure. Another component or type of reliability is homogeneity or the extent to which items on a multi-item instrument are consistent with one other. Also, equivalence reliability tells you whether multiple forms or multiple users of an instrument produce the same results.

Nurses like to know the sensitivity and specificity of screening tests. Sensitivity is the probability of getting a true positive, and specificity is the probability of getting a true negative. Prevalence of the illness in a population affects the positive and negative predictive values of a screening test.

Again, great work for completing this difficult chapter. If you are somewhat confused by these new concepts, continue to practice, practice, practice! Believe it or not, you will look back on these concepts at the end of the semester, and they will make sense.

CHAPTER 4 REVIEW QUESTIONS

1. Your test is very good at correctly identifying when a person actually has a disease. What is this is a measure of?

   a. sensitivity
   b. specificity
   c. collinearity
   d. effect size

2. If a person has a disease and tests positive for it, the result is an example of which of the following?

   a. a true negative
   b. a false positive
   c. a false negative
   d. a true positive

Questions 3–4: You are studying a new screening test. Of the 100 people who do not have a disease, 80 test negative for it with your new screen. Of the 100 people who do have the disease, 90 test positive with your screen.

3. The sensitivity of your screen is _____.
4. Your new screen's specificity is _____.

5. You have a new tool that examines outcomes in pregnancy. A previously validated tool reports that cesarean section rates in your area are 30%. The correlation between the old tool and your tool is 0.7. This result indicates which of the following?

   a. convergent validity
   b. content validity
   c. divergent validity
   d. validity from contrasting groups

Questions 6–13: You are developing a new screening test and construct the test results shown in **Figure 4-8**.

FIGURE 4-8   **A 2 × 2 Table.**

	Disease Present	**Disease Not Present**	**Totals**
Test Positive	44	3	47
Test Negative	6	97	103
Totals	50	100	150

6. How many true positives do you have?

7. Without using statistics jargon, explain what each box represents.

8. What is the sensitivity of your new test?

9. What is the specificity of your new test?

10. Give an example of a clinical situation in which this might be a good test to use.

11. What is the positive predictive value of your screening test?

12. What is the prevalence of the disease you are testing for?

13. If this disease were fatal, would you be concerned about this prevalence rate?

Research Application

Questions 14–17: A small study was done to compare the results from three different chlamydia screening tests. The results obtained are shown in **Figure 4-9**.

FIGURE 4-9	**A 2 × 2 Table for Chlamydia Screen.**

	Sensitivity	Specificity	PPV	NPV
Screen A	57	96	66	94
Screen B	85	82	37	98
Screen C	57	94	57	94

14. Which screen has the lowest specificity? Why might it still be a good screen to use?

_____

_____

15. Which screen has the highest positive predictive value? If you administered this screen in a population with a high prevalence, what would you expect to happen to the positive predictive value?

_____

_____

16. If you know that early treatment helps prevent infertility and that chlamydia is very contagious, would sensitivity or specificity be more important to you? With that in mind, which of these tests would you prefer to utilize?

_____

_____

17. If all the tests are administered in the same manner and cost the same, which one would you recommend that your clinic use? Justify your answer.

_____

_____

Questions 18–23: You are using a screening test in your clinic to detect abnormal cervical cells related to the presence of human papilloma virus (HPV). Your results are shown in **Figure 4-10**.

FIGURE 4-10 **Screen Test Results.**

	Abnormal Cells Present	Abnormal Cells Not Present	Totals
Test Positive	360	20	380
Test Negative	40	80	120
Totals	400	100	500

18. What is the prevalence of abnormal cells in your clinic? What does this mean in non-statistical language or plain English?

19. What is the sensitivity of the screen? What does this mean in non-statistical language or plain English?

20. What is the specificity of the screen? What does this mean in non-statistical language or plain English?

21. What is the positive predictive value (PPV) of the screen? What does this mean in non-statistical language or plain English?

22. What is the negative predictive value (NPV) of the screen? What does this mean in non-statistical language or plain English?

23. What is the efficacy of the screen? What does this mean in non-statistical language or plain English?

Questions 24–31: A new vaccine is developed that provides immunity to the virus causing abnormal cervical cells, and you reexamine data 2 years after the vaccine is implemented at your clinic. See the results in **Figure 4-11**.

FIGURE 4-11 **Screening Test Results After Vaccine Implementation.**

	Abnormal Cells Present	Abnormal Cells Not Present	Totals
Test Positive	180	60	240
Test Negative	20	240	260
Totals	200	300	500

24. What is the prevalence of abnormal cervical cells after the vaccine is utilized? How did the vaccine affect the prevalence?

_____

_____

25. What is the sensitivity of the screen? Does a change in prevalence affect the sensitivity?

_____

_____

26. What is the specificity of the screen? Does a change in prevalence affect the specificity?

_____

_____

27. What is the positive predictive value (PPV) of the screen? Does a change in prevalence affect the PPV? How?

_____

_____

28. What is the negative predictive value (NPV) of the screen? Does a change in prevalence affect the NPV? How?

_____

_____

29. What happens to the number of false positives when the prevalence rates go down?

_____

_____

30. What happens to the efficacy of the screen when prevalence rates go down?

_____

_____

31. Why might you consider lengthening the time between screens or developing a more specific screen with the new prevalence rate?

_____

_____

32. Melanomas are the most deadly form of skin cancer, affecting more than 53,000 Americans each year and killing more than 7,000 annually. Your state currently has 167 cases of melanoma reported and there are 1,420,000 people in the state. What is the prevalence rate in your state?

_____

_____

Questions 33–39: A clinical study is established to determine if the results of a screening stress test can be used as a predictor of the presence of heart disease. The study enrolls 100 participants who undergo a screening stress test and then have their disease state confirmed by an angiogram (gold standard). Twenty participants screened positive with their stress tests and had confirmed heart disease on their angiogram. One participant who screened positive on his stress test had a normal angiogram and did not have heart disease. Seventy-seven participants screened negative on their stress tests and had normal angiograms without heart disease.

33. Develop an appropriate 2 × 2 table illustrating this information.

34. What is the sensitivity of the screening stress test? What does this mean in non-statistical language or plain English?

35. What is the specificity of the screening stress test? What does this mean in non-statistical language or plain English?

36. What is the positive predictive value (PPV) of the screening stress test? What does this mean in English?

37. What is the negative predictive value (NPV) of the screening stress test? What does this mean in non-statistical language or plain English?

38. What is the disease prevalence in this sample?

39. What is the efficacy of this screen?

ANSWERS TO CHAPTER 4 REVIEW QUESTIONS

1. A

3. 90%

5. A

7. 44 = true positives, 3 = false positives, 47 = all positive tests, 6 = false negatives, 97 = true negatives, 103 = all negative tests, 50 = total with disease, 100 = healthy total, 150 = total population

9. 97 ÷ 100 = 97%

11. 44 ÷ 47 = 93.6%

13. Yes! A third of the population has the disease. That is a substantial disease burden.

15. A, high prevalence increases PPV; therefore, the PPV would increase.

17. Answers will vary, but should not include screen C, which has lower specificity and PPV than screen A and the same sensitivity and NPV.

19. $360 \div 400 = 90\%$ (If the patient has abnormal cervical cells, there is a 90% probability that the screen will be positive and detect the abnormal cells.)

21. $360 \div 380 = 94.7\%$ (Of all the patients who screen positive, 94.7% are patients who really have abnormal cervical cells.)

23. $440 \div 500 = 88\%$ (Eighty-eight percent of the time the screen correctly identifies the patient's disease state.)

25. $180 \div 200 = 90\%$ (stays the same)

27. $180 \div 240 = 75\%$ (PPV decreases when prevalence goes down! You are more likely to have false positives in areas with lower prevalence.)

29. False positives increase.

31. Answers will vary but should include: False positives create a financial burden because unnecessary services are provided. Also, there may be negative health impacts from the stress, anxiety, loss of work time, and any other unnecessary screens or procedures that result from the false positive screen.

33.

	Disease +	No Disease	Total
Screen test +	20	1	21
Screen test neg.	2	77	79
Total	22	78	100

35. $77/78 = 98.7\%$ When a subject does not have the disease, there is a 98.7% chance the screening test will say he or she is disease free.

37. $77/79 = 97.5\%$ When a subject has a negative screening stress test, there is a 97.5% chance he or she does not have the disease.

39. $97/100 = 97\%$

SAMPLING METHODS

DOES THE SAMPLE REPRESENT THE POPULATION?

OBJECTIVES

By the end of this chapter students will be able to:

- Compare and contrast probability and nonprobability sampling, and describe at least one example of each.

- Identify similarities and differences among simple random sampling, systematic sampling, stratified sampling, and cluster sampling.

- Identify sampling error, contrast it with sampling bias, and identify the effect of each.

- Explain why the central limit theorem is useful in statistics.

- Identify situations in which nonprobability sampling is utilized and what limits are created by doing so.

- Given a research proposal, compose inclusion and exclusion criteria.

- Evaluate sampling techniques' strengths and weakness in a current research article.

KEY TERMS

Cluster sampling
Probability sampling using a group or unit rather than an individual.

Convenience sampling
A form of nonprobability sampling that consists of collecting data from the group that is available.

Exclusion criteria
The list of characteristics that would eliminate a subject from being eligible to participate in a study.

Inclusion criteria
The list of characteristics a subject must have to be eligible to participate in a study.

Nonprobability sampling
Involves methods in which subjects do not have the same chance of being selected for participation.

Probability sampling
Techniques in which the probability of selecting each subject is known.

Quota sampling
A form of nonprobability sampling done when you select the proportions of the sample for different subgroups, much the same as in stratified sampling but without random selection.

Sampling bias
A systematic error made in the sample selection that results in a nonrandom sample.

Sampling distribution
All the possible values of a statistic from all the possible samples of a given population.

Sampling error
Differences between the sample and the population that occur due to randomization or chance.

Sampling method
The processes employed to select the subjects for a sample from the population being studied.

Simple random sampling
Probability sampling in which every subject in a population has the same chance of being selected.

Stratified sampling
Probability sampling that divides the population into subsamples according to a characteristic of interest and then randomly selects the sample from these subgroups.

Systematic sampling
Probability sampling involving the selection of subjects according to a standardized rule.

SAMPLING METHODS

Let's look at the concepts of populations and samples. A population is the whole group that is of interest to the researcher; for example, all men with heart disease are a population. However, although you are amazing as a nurse researcher, measuring the life spans of all men with heart disease is impossible. Instead, you decide to collect a representative sample of these men. To be representative of the population, the sample must reflect its important characteristics. For example, if 50% of men who have heart disease are over 60 years old, 50% of your sample population should also be men over 60 years old. Your sample, then, is a group of subjects selected from the population for the purpose of conducting your research. Because it is representative, you can then develop inferences about the original population from your sample population.

The **sampling method** you will use consists of the processes of selecting the subjects for your sample from the population under study. Of the many kinds of sampling methods, the one you select depends a great deal on your population of interest and on the options available to you at the time. There are two main kinds of sampling methods: probability sampling and nonprobability sampling.

PROBABILITY SAMPLING

Probability sampling consists of techniques in which the probability of selecting each subject is known. It can be accomplished in a number of ways, including simple random sampling, systematic sampling, stratified sampling, and cluster sampling.

SIMPLE RANDOM SAMPLING

With **simple random sampling**, every subject in a population has the same chance of being selected. Because this type of sampling requires the researcher to have access to every member of the population, it is frequently not feasible with large populations. However, suppose as the nursing researcher you wish to find out the mean age of the nurses at your hospital. You could use a list of all hospital nurses ($n = 100$) and then randomly select 50 subjects from the list for your sample. As long as selection is from all 100 nurses each time, the probability of selecting each individual is exactly the same (1/100). Although simple random sampling is the ideal, it doesn't work without access to the full population.

SYSTEMATIC SAMPLING

A similar approach, **systematic sampling**, involves selecting your subjects according to a standardized rule. One way of doing this is to number the whole population again, pick a random starting point, and then select every *n*th person. For example, you might take the same list of nurses from your hospital and randomly start with the 17th nurse on the list and then select every 9th one. When using this approach, you have to make sure the population list is not developed with any ranking order. For example, if your list is arranged by clinical track levels for each unit, the ninth person may fall into about the same track level consistently, and that may be an achievement related to age. Your sample would then not be representative of the population of nurses working at your hospital.

STRATIFIED SAMPLING

Stratified sampling divides the population into subsamples according to a characteristic of interest and then randomly selects the sample from these subgroups. The purpose is to ensure representativeness of the characteristic. An example should make that clearer. You are still trying to determine the average age of the nurses in your hospital. You are aware that 20% of the nurses have been practicing for 1 year or less, and the rest have more than 1 year of experience. You decide to use stratified random sampling to make sure your sample is representative of the population in terms of working experience. So you decide to select 20% of your sample randomly from the nurses who have 1 year or less of experience and 80% of your sample from those who have more than 1 year of experience.

CLUSTER SAMPLING

Cluster sampling uses a group or unit rather than an individual. It is used when it is difficult to find a list of the entire population. If, for example, you wanted to know the mean income of adults living in New York State, you may choose to survey everyone over age 21 in four randomly selected ZIP codes and take a weighted average score. Or, if you wanted to know the mean age of nurses employed in hospitals in New York, you may decide to randomly select a sample of hospitals in New York (each hospital is a cluster or group) and then find out the age of all of the nurses at those hospitals.

If that approach is too difficult, you can do two-staged cluster sampling. Rather than taking the age of each nurse at the cluster hospitals, you would randomly sample a group of nurses at each hospital. In effect, you randomly selected your clusters and then randomly selected your final sample from each of these clusters. Although less expensive than other methods, cluster sampling has its drawbacks in terms of statistics (greater variance), but is sometimes a necessary approach (Pagano & Gauvreau, 1993).

SAMPLING ERROR VERSUS SAMPLING BIAS

No matter which random sampling technique you choose for your study, there will always be some **sampling error**, that is, some differences between the sample and the population that occur due to chance. Anytime you are examining a random sample and not the whole population, you will encounter some differences that are not under your control and that occur due only to the randomization or chance.

Sampling error, however, is not the same as **sampling bias**, which is a systematic error

made in the sample selection that results in a nonrandom sample. In the previous example, you decided to take a systematic sample from a list of nurses at your hospital to determine the mean number of years they worked at your hospital. Unfortunately, you did not realize that the list was arranged by clinical track levels for each unit. You chose to start at the beginning and sample every ninth person. Unfortunately, the ninth person fell in about the same track level consistently, and track levels are related to the number of years worked at the hospital. Your results had a significant amount of sampling bias and were not representative of the population of interest.

SAMPLING DISTRIBUTIONS

Talking about the benefits of random sampling can get a little statistical, but bear with me. Suppose you collect a random sample of nurses from a population of nurses, calculate the mean age, and keep doing this with other random samples of nurses from the same population. Eventually you will develop a distribution of the mean age. This is your **sampling distribution**, which consists of all the possible values of a statistic from all the possible samples of a given population (Corty, 2007). See **Figures 5-1** and **5-2**.

The really useful thing about sampling distributions is that if your sample size is large enough (usually at least greater than 30, some say 50), the distribution of the sample means is always normally distributed even if the original population is not (Sullivan, 2007). You can thank the central limit theorem. For the purposes of this text, you don't need to delve too much into the explanation. The takeaway message is that, when a population is not distributed normally, it takes a lot more work to analyze.

FIGURE 5-1	**Sampling Distribution for the Mean Age of Nurses.**

Sample	Mean Age
One	28
Two	30
Three	30
Four	30
Five	28
Six	26
Seven	32
Eight	32
Nine	34

FIGURE 5-2	**Graph of Sample Distribution of Mean Age From Nine Samples.**

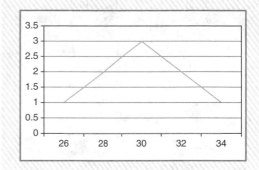

FROM THE STATISTICIAN   *BrendanHeavey*

The Central Limit Theorem and Standardized Scores

The central limit theorem is your friend. It makes a lot of analyses a lot simpler. It is a little tough to grasp perhaps, but, if you apply yourself just a little bit, you will be able to pick it up without a problem. Then you can apply it later on anytime you want.

One way to understand the central limit theorem is to see what happens when you roll a bunch of 10-sided dice. You can apply this analogy to any random experiment that involves identically likely outcomes.

If we were to roll a 10-sided die 1,000 times and plot a histogram of your results, the graph could look something like the one in **Figure 5-3**. We could get a huge amount of possible bar charts, but they would all look something like the one in the figure. In fact, in the long run this experiment would use what we call the *uniform distribution* because all cases are equally likely. If we were to roll a single die 1,000, 2,000, or even 10,000 times, all the bars would still look approximately the same.

Now let's think about what would happen if we were to use two 10-sided dice, roll them 1,000 times, and calculate the average value shown on the faces. It just so happens I enjoy doing this sort of thing in my spare time, so I went ahead and did so. The result is shown in **Figure 5-4**. What do you notice? The bars tend to look more bell shaped, don't they? There were a whole lot more results between 4 and 6 than there were 1s and 10s. When you roll two dice, there are a lot

(continues)

FROM THE STATISTICIAN *Brendan Heavey*

more ways to get an average between 4 and 6 than there are to get a 1 or a 10. In fact, the only way to average a 1 is by having both dice come up with 1s.

Now let's look at what happens when we use six 10-sided dice and take the average. The bar graph in **Figure 5-5** looks even more bell shaped.

This progression demonstrates the central limit theory. In fact, what the underlying distributions look like doesn't matter; you could use a 4-sided die, a 12-sided die, a 6-sided die, or a 20-sided die and plot the outcomes. As you take more and more samples, the resulting distribution of the averages of all the dice will tend to look more and more bell shaped.

Remember that we're talking about the mean value of all the rolls. You can't just roll a single die a million times and expect it to look more and more bell shaped as you increase the number of rolls. You have to look at the mean value across multiple experiments.

The central limit theorem is one of the most important in all of statistics. It can be proven, but it takes a whole lot of math that I'm sure you don't want to see. We can make some very important and very interesting deductions from this theorem, however. One is that, when you take a sample in any experiment, the population variables can be distributed in any matter you want, but the mean of the sample measurement will always be distributed as a normal distribution in the long run. This becomes really important when we compare the means of two samples. (Curb your enthusiasm! I know I can't wait!)

FIGURE 5-3   **Central Limit Theorem: One 10-Sided Die Rolled 1,000 Times.**

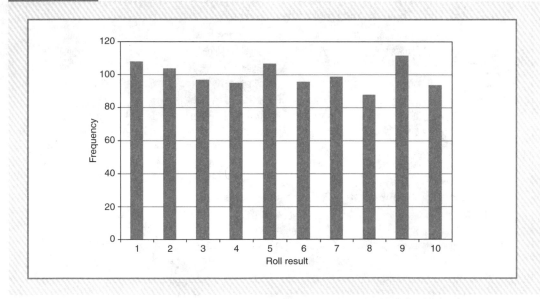

FIGURE 5-4   **Central Limit Theorem: Two 10-Sided Dice Rolled 1,000 Times and Averaged.**

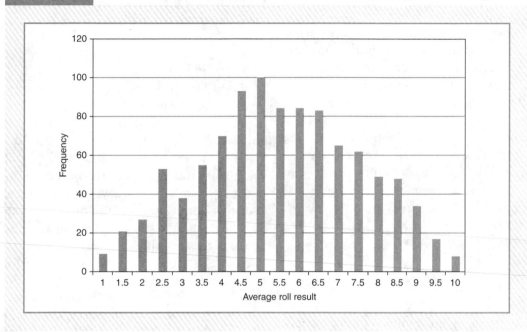

FIGURE 5-5   **Central Limit Theorem: Six 10-Sided Dice Rolled 1,000 Times and Averaged.**

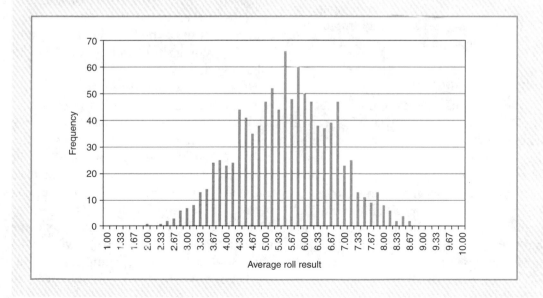

NONPROBABILITY SAMPLING

The reality of research is that it has budgetary and time limits. In these situations, sometimes nonprobability sampling methods are necessary or simply more practical. **Nonprobability sampling** consists of methods in which subjects do not have the same chance of being selected for participation. It is *not randomized*. When you are reading nursing research, never assume a sample was randomly selected. You need to identify how the sample was selected before you can tell whether the claims the research makes are valid or what their limitations may be.

TYPES OF NONPROBABILITY SAMPLING

There are many different ways nonprobability sampling can be used in both quantitative and qualitative research. Two of the most popular methods for quantitative research are convenience sampling and quota sampling, whereas qualitative research may employ network sampling or purposive sampling.

Convenience Sampling

The most popular form of nonprobability sampling in healthcare research is **convenience sampling**, which is simply collecting data from the available group. For example, suppose you were trying to determine the mean age of the nurses in your hospital. You go to the oncology unit and ask all the nurses working that shift their age. You would be taking a convenience sample. Convenience samples are usually relatively quick and inexpensive, but they may not be

representative of the population and therefore limit any inferences you may choose to make about the population.

Quota Sampling

In **quota sampling**, you select the proportions of the sample for different subgroups, as in stratified sampling. For example, if 50% of your population works day shift, 30% works evening shift, and 20% works night shift, your sample will have those same proportions. I bet right now you are thinking, "But this doesn't seem to be different from stratified random sampling." Well, so far— you're right, nothing is different yet. The difference is after this point. If you need a final sample size of 100, with stratified random sampling, you would *randomly* select 50 subjects from day shift workers, 30 from evening shift workers, and 20 from night shift workers. Quota sampling, on the other hand, is nonprobability sampling so it is not randomized. After you decide on the proportions of the sample, you collect subjects continuously until you have 50 day shift subjects, 30 evening shift subjects, and 20 night shift subjects.

Now suppose that you decide to collect this sample at 3:30 in the lobby of your hospital. Everyone who participates gets a free coffee coupon. Fifty day shift nurses participate on their way out, and 30 evening shift nurses participated on their way in. You have enrolled all your day and evening nurses but are still waiting for the night nurses. At 10:45 the night shift nurses start to come through the lobby. As you are surveying the night shift staffers, an evening nurse, ending her shift, comes over and volunteers to participate. You cannot include her because you already have your quota of evening shift nurses and are still collecting only night shift nurses. The evening shift nurse becomes irate because she really wants to be in your study (read "really wants the coffee"), and she calls several of her friends to also come in and volunteer. (Nurses *will* do a lot for free coffee.) They, too, are upset because they were not working that day and were therefore never given the opportunity to participate. Because they worked the day and evening shifts, they are also not eligible to participate because you have already filled the quotas for these shifts.

You end up sitting in the lobby with several very upset day and evening nurses who don't understand why you can't let them participate, at the same time still asking the night shift nurses to join the study and giving them coffee. "The night shift gets everything!" the other nurses complain. Because you are exceptionally patient and have already had your extra coffee that day, you patiently explain that quota sampling does not give the same opportunity to everyone to participate. You are very sorry. You would love to give everyone free coffee, but you need only night nurses now. This is how quota sampling works. Once you have reached the quota for that particular group, no matter how many more subjects from that group arrive you do not enroll them and only collect data from the groups for which you have not met your quota.

Of course, after such a stressful experience you may also decide either to change your sampling method or to go to a different hospital to collect data next time. These nurses are intense!

NONPROBABILITY SAMPLING IN QUALITATIVE RESEARCH

Many other nonprobability-based sampling methods are more frequently used with qualitative research. Network sampling, for example, utilizes the social networks of friends and families to gather information. This technique is frequently used when you need information about groups that hesitate to participate in research, such as youth gangs. Another technique, purposive sampling, includes subjects because they have particularly strong bases of information. You may decide to use network sampling to study youth gangs after you are able to gain the trust and support of a gang leader. She then refers other members of her gang to you, and you are able eventually to speak to a group of 10 youth gang members. You may then decide to collect a purposive sample (specific individuals are selected to participate because of the information they are able to contribute) and further study three of these young women because they are lifelong gang members and can give you the greatest insight into the characteristics and behaviors you are studying.

INCLUSION AND EXCLUSION CRITERIA

No matter which sampling method you select, as the researcher you need to develop sample inclusion and exclusion criteria.

- **Inclusion criteria** make up the list of characteristics a subject must have to be eligible to participate in your study. These criteria identify the target population and limit the generalizability of your study results to this population.

For example, if you are studying the effect of taking a multivitamin on future prostate cancer development, the foremost inclusion criterion is male gender. (Only men have prostates so it would be pointless to include women in this study.)

- **Exclusion criteria** are the criteria or characteristics that eliminate a subject from being eligible to participate in your study. Exclusion criteria frequently include the current or past presence of the outcome of interest. For example, in your study about the vitamin-mediated prevention of prostate cancer, having prostate cancer would be one of your exclusion criteria. If the subject already has or has had the disease, you can't determine whether the vitamin helps to prevent it.

SUMMARY

That was a lot of information to take in for one chapter, so take a deep breath and allow your brain to slow down. Let's highlight the main ideas.

A sampling method consists of the processes that help you pick the subjects for your sample from the population you are interested in studying. The two main kinds of sampling methods are probability sampling and nonprobability sampling. Probability sampling involves techniques in which the probability of selecting each subject is known. The types of probability sampling include simple random sampling, systematic sampling, stratified sampling, and cluster sampling. Nonprobability sampling involves methods in which subjects do not have the same chance of being selected for participation. In other words, sampling is not randomized. Nonprobability sampling includes convenience sampling, quota sampling, network sampling, and purposive sampling.

When you are collecting samples, sampling error can occur; that is, some differences between the sample and the population always occur due to randomization or chance. Sampling bias, however, can also occur, which is the result of a systematic error in the sample selection, rendering it nonrandom.

Finally, all research studies have inclusion and exclusion criteria. Inclusion criteria make up a list of characteristics that a subject must have to participate in your study. Exclusion criteria are the criteria or characteristics that eliminate a subject from being eligible to participate.

You are done with this chapter. Take a break. Drink some tea and unwind a bit. You've earned a break!

CHAPTER 5 REVIEW QUESTIONS

1. What is the difference between probability and nonprobability sampling?

2. Identify whether probability or nonprobability sampling was utilized for each entry in the following list:
   a. Convenience sampling
   b. Cluster sampling

    c. Simple random sampling

    d. Quota sampling

    e. Systematic sampling

    f. Stratified sampling

3. What is the difference between sampling error and sampling bias? Which one is very concerning to researchers?

Research Application

> **Questions 4–5:** One study used a convenience sample drawn from clients utilizing two community-based obstetric offices in an area with limited socioeconomic conditions. The sample was drawn largely from the community surrounding the offices, and the findings may not be generalizable to this population or other populations that differ significantly from this sample.[*]

4. Why should a reader be careful about developing inferences about the population of interest from the article?

5. How could the researcher have designed this study differently so that developing inferences about the population of interest would be less of a concern?

6. Hemoglobin levels are usually 12–16 g/100 mL for women and 14–18 g/100 mL for men. If you have a sampling distribution of mean hemoglobin levels (collected from 60 hospitals) with a mean of 16 g/100 mL and a standard deviation of 2 g/100 mL, calculate the range of hemoglobin levels that would include 68% of your sample means.

7. What percentage of sample means would fall between 12 g/100 mL and 20 g/100 mL?

8. If one of the hospitals in your sample was a Veterans Affairs facility with 97% male patients, would you expect the mean hemoglobin level collected only from the patients at that hospital to be any different from those of other hospitals?

9. If one of the hospitals in your sample was the regional Women's and Children's Hospital, would you expect the mean hemoglobin level collected at that hospital to be different from that of the other hospitals?

10. You would like to compare the wait time at your clinic this year versus last year. Your electronic medical record database contains the check-in time and rooming time for all patients seen in the last 2 years. You import the data into your SPSS statistics program and program the computer to randomly select 500 patients seen last year and 500 patients seen this year. What type of sample is this? Is it a probability or nonprobability sampling method?

11. You decide to start again, this time programing SPSS to select every 14th patient each year. What type of sample is this? Is it a probability or nonprobability sample?

---

*This text is reprinted with the permission of Elsevier and was originally published in Heavey, E., Moysich, K., Hyland, A., Druschel, C., & Sill, M. (2008). Female adolescents' perception of male partners' pregnancy desire. *Journal of Midwifery and Women's Health, 53*(4), 338–344. Copyright Elsevier (2008).

12. A researcher examining drinking patterns in his county distributes his survey at a bar on the first Friday of three consecutive months. What type of sample is this? Is it a probability or nonprobability sample?

13. The researcher decides he wants his sample of 200 to be 50% female and distributes his survey at the bar to the first 100 women who arrive and the first 100 men who arrive. This is what type of sample? Is it a probability or nonprobability sample?

14. You would like to know the average wait time of adult patients seen in federally funded health clinics in the United States. You randomly select 100 clinics and then collect the wait time for 100 randomly selected patient visits. What type of sample is this? Is it a probability or nonprobability sample?

15. You conduct a well-designed study involving a random sample. Your analysis shows this sample is normally distributed and representative of the population; however, the mean age in the sample is 29.4 years and the mean age in the population is 30 years. What is this type of difference called, and what is the likely cause of the difference? Should the researcher be concerned?

16. A researcher wants to examine drinking patterns in men and women in bars in New York State. She randomly selects five bars and then randomly selects subjects at those bars to complete her surveys on four randomly selected weekends. However, she did not realize that two of the five bars selected were for gay men and another bar was having a draft special for the football playoff games for three of the four weekends. Her sample ends up being 85% male whereas the population who attends bars is only 65% male. Is this sample representative? Why or why not? Would this be an example of sample error or sample bias? Should the researcher be concerned?

Questions 17–20: You would like to ensure your sample is representative of the racial mix seen in your population of interest. The population is 50% Asian, 20% African American, 20% Caucasian, and 10% other. You need a sample of 500 subjects. You program SPSS to randomly select 250 Asian subjects from your population, 100 African American subjects, 100 Caucasian subjects, and 50 subjects identified as other.

17. What type of sample is this? Is it a probability or nonprobability sample?

18. You are interested in how race may impact total cholesterol. Your study classifies race in the above categories. What level of measurement is this variable?

19. What is your dependent variable?

20. Your sample is normally distributed with an average total cholesterol of 211 and a standard deviation of 7. In what range would you expect the total cholesterol to be for 68% of your sample?

Questions 21–25: The nurse researcher is studying the impact of social media usage on the quality of adolescent relationships. She identifies 22 teen subjects and asks about whom they contact on Facebook, via Twitter, and via text messaging. She then follows up with an interview with those who have the most contacts and examines these relationships further.

21. What is the independent variable in this study?

22. What is the dependent variable in this study?

23. If the quality of adolescent relationships is reported as poor, good, or excellent, what level variable is this?

24. If instead the researcher asks these adolescents to rank the quality of their relationships on a scale of 0–10, what level of measurement would this variable be?

25. What type of sampling method is this? Is it probability or nonprobability sampling?

Questions 26–30: You conduct a well-designed study involving a random sample ($n = 84$). Age is measured in years. Your analysis shows that in this sample age is normally distributed and representative of the population. The youngest subjects are 15 ($n = 2$), one subject is 16, and the oldest subject is 46 years old; the mean age is 29.4 years and there is a standard deviation of 3 years.

26. What is the median age in this sample?

27. What age range would include 95% of the subjects in your sample?

28. What is the age range of the sample?

29. What percentage of your sample is 15 years of age or less?

30. If age is measured as 15–20 years, 25–35 years, and >35 years, what level of measurement is this variable?

31. If a variable is measured as eligible to vote and not eligible to vote, what level of measurement is this variable?

32. If you randomly select 250 individuals who are on a voter registration list and 72 report they will vote for an independent candidate, what percentage is planning to vote for an independent candidate?

Questions 33–35: You decide to interview all college athletic team captains at three state universities because of their direct knowledge of team initiation activities and hazing practices.

33. What type of sample is this? Is it a probability or nonprobability sampling method?

34. Your subjects must have been team captains for at least 3 months, on a Division I university–affiliated sports team, who are eligible to play in the upcoming season. These subject characteristics are examples of what?

35. Team captains currently on the injured or inactive list are not eligible to participate in the study. This is an example of what?

ANSWERS TO CHAPTER 5 REVIEW QUESTIONS

1. With probability sampling, the probability of selecting each subject is known and is the same. With nonprobability sampling, the subjects do not have the same chance of being selected.

3. Sampling error is random error due to chance. Systematic error results in a nonrandom sample and is very concerning to researchers.

5. A randomized sample improves representativeness and expands generalizability.

7. 95% (mean 16 +/− two standard deviations)

9. Yes, hemoglobin levels are lower for women and children.

11. Systematic sample, probability sample

13. Convenience sample with quota sampling, nonprobability

15. A sampling error likely due to chance or randomization; the researcher does not have to be concerned.

17. Stratified, probability sample

19. Total cholesterol

21. Social media use

23. Ordinal

25. Network sampling, nonprobability

27. 23.4–35.4 years

29. $2/84 = 2.4\%$

31. Nominal

33. Purposeful sample, nonprobability sampling

35. Exclusion criteria

GENERATING THE RESEARCH IDEA

WHAT IS MY RESEARCH IDEA?

By the end of this chapter students will be able to:

- State the null hypothesis.
- Define an alternative hypothesis.
- Describe hypothesis testing.
- Compare rejecting the null hypothesis and failing to reject the null hypothesis.
- Correlate alpha, the chance of a type one error, and statistical significance.
- Identify a type one error, and propose one method to avoid it.

- Distinguish between statistically significant results and nonsignificant results in a current research article.
- Debate clinical significance given a research article with statistical significance present.
- Analyze statistical information to determine whether statistical significance is present.

KEY TERMS

Alpha (a)
The significance level, usually 0.05. The probability of incorrectly rejecting the null hypothesis or making a type one error.

Alternative hypothesis
Usually the relationship or association or difference that the researcher actually believes to be present.

Clinically significant
A result that is statistically significant and clinically useful.

Fail to reject the null hypothesis
When you do not have enough statistical strength to show a difference or an association.

Hypothesis
An observation or idea that can be tested.

Hypothesis testing
The application of a statistical test to determine whether an observation or idea is to be refuted or accepted.

Null hypothesis
There is no difference or association between variables that is any greater or less than would be expected by chance.

Reject the null hypothesis
When you have enough statistical strength to show a difference or an association.

Statistical significance
When the difference you observe between two samples is large enough that it is not simply due to chance.

Type one error
Occurs when you incorrectly reject the null hypothesis.

HYPOTHESIS TESTING

When you arrive at the clinic at 8 a.m., you are prepared to administer the flu vaccine to patients who show up for one. Already people are waiting, and many are wearing business attire. The turnout is much higher than your clinic expected, processing everyone is taking longer than expected, and you are the only nurse. The patients are brought into a central receiving area, their background information is collected, and then they come to your station for the actual injection. After the first hour you notice that most of your patients are elderly or unemployed. You realize that it is after now after 9 a.m. Very few individuals who report outside employment arrive during the hours of 9 a.m. and 5 p.m. You start to wonder whether employed individuals are less likely to get their flu shots because they are unable to come to the clinic during standard business hours, and those who arrived before work may not have been able to stay due to the long delays.

This is a **hypothesis**, an observation or idea that can be tested. You decide to determine whether your observation is actually true. First, you develop your **null hypothesis**, which states that there is no difference or association between variables that is any greater or less than would be expected by chance. (The null hypothesis is represented as H_0.) In this case, the null hypothesis is that there is no relationship between employment status and having a flu shot at your clinic. The **alternative hypothesis** is usually the relationship or association or difference that the researcher actually believes to be present. (The alternative hypothesis is represented as H_1.) In this case, your alternative hypothesis is that those who are employed are less likely to get a flu shot at your clinic. **Hypothesis testing**, a big fancy term for figuring out whether you are right, involves using a statistical test to determine whether your hypothesis is true. In this case, that night when the clinic closes, you decide to collect the information that was gathered on all the patients who arrived at the clinic from 8 a.m. until 9 p.m. that week. This is your sample.

Your statistical analysis of the sample enables you to do one of two things:

- If the trend of having very few employed patients arriving for flu shots at your clinic continued throughout the day, you may find a statistically significant difference (we'll tell you how to do this later in the chapter) between the number of employed people who received the flu shot at your clinic that week and those who were not employed. You are then in a position to **reject the null hypothesis**. You have determined the difference between the two groups is greater than the difference you might expect to result from chance. You have evidence of a statistically significant relationship between employment status and receiving a flu shot at your clinic, and you have demonstrated support for your alternative hypothesis.
- On the other hand, let's say you collect and analyze the data from the whole week and find that, although there were fewer employed people receiving flu shots between 9 a.m. and 5 p.m. (your initial impression), between 8 and 9 a.m. and between 5 and 9 p.m. most of the flu

shot recipients were employed. In this case, your statistical analysis may not show a significant difference between the number of people who received the flu shot who were employed and those who were not. You would then **fail to reject the null hypothesis**. This is the important point: You can never "accept" or "prove" the null hypothesis, which is the absence of something. You can only "disprove" it (reject it) or "fail to disprove" it (fail to reject it).

Here's an analogy for this slightly confusing concept that obstetrics nurses usually understand fairly quickly, so let's use their clinical experience to help you, too. When a pregnant patient has an ultrasound, the technician attempts to determine the sex of the infant by detecting the presence of a penis. The null hypothesis is that there is no penis. The alternative hypothesis is that there is one. If a penis is detected, the ultrasound technician can state that there is one and the baby is a boy. If a penis is not detected, the technician cannot be sure that there isn't one; it might be present but undetected (Corty, 2007). As a nurse–midwife, I frequently explained to my patients that if the ultrasound technician told them they are carrying a baby boy, they could consider the report fairly reliable (but notice this is still not a probability of 100%). However, I have been in the delivery room when a predicted girl turned out to be a bashful boy. Never overstate what your data allows you to say! You can never say for sure that something does not exist, but the mere presence of what you are looking for can demonstrate that it does. That being said, it is also important to remember that statistics is all about probability, and there is always a possibility of an error so you can never "prove" anything with absolute certainty. The technician who thinks she sees a baby boy could still just be wrong.

STATISTICAL SIGNIFICANCE

Statistical significance means that the difference you observe between two samples is large enough that it is not simply due to chance. Statistical significance is a key concept. There are many different ways to show statistical significance, but the basic idea remains the same: If you take two or more representative samples from the same population, you would expect to find approximately the same difference again and again. If you have a statistically significant result, you can reject the null hypothesis.

But how do you know whether your result is statistically significant? At the beginning of the study, the researcher selects the significance level, or **alpha**, which is usually 0.05. This number is simply the probability assigned to incorrectly rejecting the null hypothesis, or to making what is called a **type one error**. For example, you conduct a study examining the association between eating a high-fiber breakfast and 10 a.m. serum glucose levels. The null hypothesis is that a high-fiber breakfast is not associated with the 10 a.m. serum glucose levels. The alternative is that it is. You select an alpha of 0.05, which means you are accepting that there is a 5% chance that you will reject the null hypothesis incorrectly and report that eating a high-fiber breakfast is associated with a change in blood sugar levels at 10 a.m. when in actuality it is not.

The alpha is therefore the chance of reporting a statistically significant difference that does not exist. An alpha of 0.05 can also be interpreted to mean that you are 95% sure that the significant difference you are reporting is correct.

Corresponding to the alpha (which is represented by α) is what statisticians call the p-value, the probability of observing a value of a test statistic if the null hypothesis (there is no relationship, association, or difference between the variables) is true. In other words, a p-value tells you the probability of finding your test statistic if there is no relationship between the variables. This is also the probability that an observed relationship, association, or difference is just due to chance. For example, if your study examining the consumption of a high-fiber breakfast and 10 a.m. glucose levels has a test statistic with a p-value of 0.03, then the probability that the observations in your study would occur if there was no relationship between these variables (or by chance) is only 3%. This means you are 97% sure that the variables in your study do have a relationship. If your study has an alpha of 0.05 it means you accept up to a 5% chance of making a type one error and reporting that a relationship exists when it is just by chance. If your test statistic shows you have only a 3% chance of making a type one error, then you can confidently reject the null hypothesis and state there is a relationship, an association, or a difference between the variables. If the p-value is less than the alpha, the researcher should reject the null hypothesis. If it is greater, the chance of making a type one error is too great, and the researcher must fail to reject the null hypothesis. Subtracting the p-value from 1 tells you how sure the researcher is about rejecting the null hypothesis (e.g., a p-value of 0.03 means the researcher is 97% sure that the observed relationship is not just due to chance).

FROM THE STATISTICIAN *Brendan Heavey*

Alpha of 0.05: Standard Convention versus Experiment Specific

Interpreting *p*-values can be a science in and of itself. Let me share with you how I think of *p*-values.

Think about your favorite courtroom drama. Whether you recall O.J. Simpson's trial, *A Few Good Men*, *To Kill a Mockingbird*, or *Erin Brockovich*, in all these situations, the defendants are innocent until proven guilty. Therefore, the null hypothesis in these "experiments" is that the defendant is innocent. At all these trials, a defendant is declared not guilty, never innocent. The trial is being conducted—like an experiment—to determine whether to reject the null hypothesis. The null hypothesis cannot be proven; it can only be disproven.

In O.J.'s case, a lot of people thought there was enough evidence to reject the null hypothesis of innocence and find him guilty. However, as in any criminal case, O.J. had to be declared guilty beyond a reasonable doubt. This is a very stringent criterion. Later, in the civil case, the district attorney only had to show a preponderance of evidence to have him declared guilty, which was a much easier task. So O.J. was found not guilty in the criminal trial, but guilty in the civil trial. This split decision is the equivalent of different alpha levels determining statistical significance in statistical experiments. The courts reduced the stringency of the test to determine guilt by reducing the burden of proof necessary to convict in a civil trial. Scientists can do the same thing in statistical tests by increasing alpha (which "decreases the burden of proof" in your study). Notice that showing a defendant is guilty in a civil trial (due to a preponderance of evidence) is easier to do than showing he or she is guilty in a criminal trial (beyond a reasonable doubt). Think of a statistical test the same way. If your *p*-value is 0.07 you would reject the null hypothesis if your alpha is 0.10 (less stringent) but not if your alpha is 0.05 (more stringent). It is easier to reject the null hypothesis at the 0.10 level than the 0.05 level.

Note that 0.05 is a very arbitrary alpha cutoff. It has persisted to this day only because R.A. Fisher preferred it, and he's one of the most important statisticians and scientists of all time. He started the practice back in the 1920s, and it has stuck ever since. However, at times scientists use a more stringent cutoff of 0.01 or a less stringent one of 0.1. It is a sliding scale to determine statistical significance, just like the sliding scale of burden of proof in the courtroom.

STATISTICAL SIGNIFICANCE VERSUS CLINICAL SIGNIFICANCE

Statistically significant differences are not the same as **clinically significant** differences. Clinically significant differences are large enough to indicate a preferential course of treatment or a difference in clinical approach to patient care. To be clinically significant, a result must be statistically significant and clinically useful. Results that are statistically significant are not necessarily clinically significant, which is a more subjective conclusion.

For example, as a nurse manager, you are approached by the largest chocolate sales team in your region. They say that the newest research shows that patients who receive free chocolate from the hospital are discharged earlier. Well, you might be interested in reading the study. The chocolate team conducted a study with 700,000 participants and found that those who were given free chocolate went home on average 2 minutes earlier than those who didn't. Although you know chocolate makes people feel better, you do not see these statistically significant results as being clinically significant because a saving of 2 minutes has very little impact on your unit. Besides, what do the follow-up studies say about tooth decay? (In addition, having a very large sample size [700,000 people] in a study might result in statistical significance even though the difference found [the effect size] is actually very small.)

FROM THE STATISTICIAN *Brendan Heavey*

Statistical Testing

What if we want to use the information we collect to make informed decisions? What if we want to use the data to decide how to treat patients or how to predict who will most benefit from new treatments? Questions like these make up the core of hypothesis testing. This "From the Statistician" is a little more difficult, but it is at the very heart of the statistical science presented in this text, so try to hang in there with me.

Most statistical testing procedures can be broken down into the five steps shown in **Figure 6-1**. A hypothesis test is like a funnel that sorts a whole bunch of information in the form of sample data and decision rules and then spits out a single, easy-to-understand *p*-value. Isn't it great that there is an easy-to-understand answer after all that work?!

FIGURE 6-1   **Hypothesis Testing Steps.**

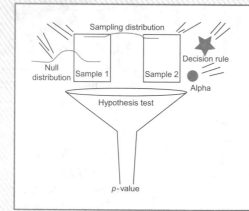

1. State the null and alternative hypotheses.
2. *Significance level:* Determine which alpha to use to determine statistical significance.
3. *Statistical test:* Determine which statistical test to use.
4. Compare the distribution of the statistic computed in step 3 to the distribution under the null hypothesis and report a *p*-value.
5. *Decision rule:* Decide whether to reject the null hypothesis or not. (Is the sample distribution different enough from the null distribution to say it is more than a chance occurrence?)

The first two steps in a hypothesis test are relatively straightforward, and you already know how to do them. First, you state your null and alternative hypotheses; then you pick the significance level (alpha) that you wish to have in your study. Typically, the alpha is 0.05, which means that, if you find a difference, you are 95% sure it is truly there, not just a chance occurrence.

The p-value is related to the alpha. It is just a probability statement about the research. Just as probability ranges between 0 and 1, so do p-values. The closer a p-value gets to 1, the more likely the related event is (in this case, the conclusion). The closer the p-value gets to 0, the less likely it is. Piece of cake, right?

Choosing which statistical test to perform is more difficult. Which test you choose depends on a number of things, but usually the most important are how many samples will be compared, how many parts of the population will be estimated, and the format of the variables.

The different forms of statistical tests have a lot in common, though, so we can speak about them in general terms. Many tests involve computing a so-called "test statistic." One type of test statistic is a Z-score, which is simply a test statistic that is a standardized measure in a normal distribution. A Z-score tells you how many standard deviations the observation is from the mean. For example, if $Z = 3.4$, the observation is 3.4 standard deviations above the mean score. If $Z = -0.2$, then the observation is 0.2 standard deviations below the mean score. A Z-score, like any other test statistic you compute, has a corresponding p-value, which is then used to make the decision to reject or fail to reject the null hypothesis. But where do these p-values come from?

Figure 6-2 is a picture of a prototypical hypothesis test using the normal distribution. We can see that the area under the normal curve varies when drawing vertical lines at different Z-scores. This area is what we need to know in order to report p-values. In this case, 2.5% of the probability can be found in each tail of the distribution. The area underneath the normal curve, above the horizontal axis and to the outside of our vertical lines, totals 0.05 (0.025 in each tail). These vertical lines represent the Z-value that corresponds with these probability levels. In this case, the Z-value of 2 or 22 is greater than 1.96 (the cutoff for statistical significance on the horizontal axis), so our statistical test falls in the upper tail of the null distribution. Whenever that happens, we say that the observed data is significantly different from what we would expect under the null distribution. Therefore, we conclude this observed difference is not

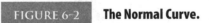

| FIGURE 6-2 | **The Normal Curve.** |

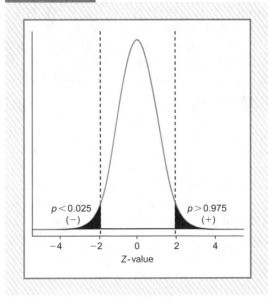

just due to sampling error or chance, and we reject the null hypothesis.

So you should be able to figure out the big question: How much area is under the whole curve in the normal distribution? The answer is 1 or 100% of the probability. As your observation gets farther and farther away from the mean, two things happen:

- The Z-score gets pushed farther and farther into the tails of the statistical distribution.
- The p-value associated with that Z-score gets smaller and smaller.

And, as you already know, the smaller the p-value is, the less likely it is that this observation is just due to chance and the more sure you are that the difference you found is actually there. You should now be able to understand the link between Z-scores and p-values. This concept directly transfers from Z-scores and other scores such as T-scores, F-scores, and chi-squared scores. Those tests differ in the types of data involved as well as in the quantities being estimated, but they work on this same principle. If the p-value associated with the computed test statistic is less than the alpha value chosen in the decision rule, we should reject the null hypothesis.

SUMMARY

You have just completed Chapter 6! The concepts are getting more technical, but keep reviewing and practicing to maintain and enhance your knowledge. Now we can review some of the important concepts in this chapter.

A hypothesis is an observation or idea that can be tested. The null hypothesis states that there is no relationship, association, or difference. The alternative hypothesis is the opposite of the null: There is a relationship, association, or difference (what you actually think is true). Hypothesis testing involves using a sample to determine whether your hypothesis is true.

When you reject the null hypothesis, you have found statistical support for your alternative hypothesis. When you fail to reject the null hypothesis, you do not have enough statistical strength to say there is a relationship or an association. There may not really be a relationship, or you may not have a sample that is large enough. You can never accept the null hypothesis. If you reject the null hypothesis incorrectly, it is a type one error.

Statistical significance means that the difference you observed between two samples is large enough that it is not simply due to chance. To determine statistical significance, you need to identify a significance level, called the alpha, which is usually 0.05. If your p-value is less than alpha, you have statistical significance. For something to be clinically significant, a result must be statistically significant and clinically useful.

This chapter presented a lot of information, but if you are able to grasp these concepts, you are doing well! If it still seems a bit murky don't worry. We will continue to work with these ideas and reinforce them as you build your knowledge!

CHAPTER 6 REVIEW QUESTIONS

1. You are conducting a study to determine whether there is an association between years worked in nursing and salary earned. Write the null and alternative hypotheses.

2. If you find a *p*-value of 0.09, what would you conclude?

3. If you find a *p*-value of 0.03, what would you conclude?

4. If you reject the null hypothesis, what type of error is it if you are wrong?

5. If your *p*-value is 0.03, is the conclusion clinically significant?

6. You are conducting a study to determine whether there is an association between a positive toxicology screen for Rohypnol (flunitrazepam) and signs of sexual assault in a sample collected from three large emergency rooms throughout your state. Write the null and alternative hypotheses.

7. As the primary investigator in this study, you realize your results may be utilized in a courtroom setting, and you do not want to make a type one error. Would you prefer an alpha of 0.05, 0.10, or 0.01?

8. Your study includes all individuals who arrive in the three emergency rooms with a diagnosis of sexual assault over a 1-month period. This is what type of sample?

9. You conduct the study with an alpha of 0.05, and your test statistic has a *p*-value of 0.02. What do you conclude?

10. You get the consent of the study participants and conduct a follow-up study in which you interview the family members of the individuals included in your study. This is an example of what type of sampling?

11. You ask the family members to describe the appearance and the manner of the individuals who were assaulted when they were taken to the emergency room. Is this a qualitative or quantitative measurement?

12. You also collect a measure of the patient's sedation provided by the sexual assault nurse examiner. It is on a 5-point scale: 0 for no sedation, 1 for mild sedation, 2 for moderate sedation, 3 for heavy sedation, and 5 for unable to arouse. What level of measurement is this?

_____

_____

13. In your sample of 45 patients, 10 showed no signs of sedation, 12 were mildly sedated, 3 were moderately sedated, 13 were heavily sedated, and 7 were not arousable. What percentage were mild or moderately sedated?

_____

14. What is the median level of sedation?

_____

15. You are putting together a grouped frequencies table and want to categorize these responses as patients showing signs of sedation and those not showing signs of sedation. How many patients showed signs of sedation? What percentage of your sample is this?

_____

_____

Questions 16–40: A researcher believes there is risk between the strain of human papillomavirus (HPV) infection and the risk of cervical cell abnormalities.

16. Write an appropriate null hypothesis.

_____

17. Write an appropriate alternative hypothesis.

_____

18. If HPV infection is measured as not infected, infected with a low-risk strain, or infected with a high-risk strain, what level of measurement is this variable?

_____

19. If the presence of cervical cell abnormalities are measured as biopsy results positive or negative, what level of measurement is this variable?

_____

20. If cervical cell abnormalities are measured as biopsy pathology results of negative, CIN I, CIN II, CIN III, or Cancer in Situ (these are progressively worse levels of abnormality), what level of measurement is the variable?

_____

21. In the population, 30% of cervical biopsies are negative, 40% are CIN I, 20% are CIN II, 5% are CIN III, and 5% are Cancer in Situ (CIS). A random selection of hospitals is made and a random selection of biopsy results is reviewed. What type of sample is this?

_____

_____

22. Is it a probability or nonprobability sample?

_____

_____

23. In the random sample of 120 biopsies, 16 are negative, 42 are CIN I, 30 are CIN II, 22 are CIN III, and 10 are CIS. In the same sample, 1 person is HPV negative, 87 are HPV positive with the low-risk strain, and 32 are HPV positive with the high-risk strain. What percentage of your sample are CIN II or greater?

_____

24. What percentage are not infected with a high-risk strain?

_____

25. What percentage have an abnormal cervical biopsy?

_____

26. What is the median biopsy result?

_____

27. What biopsy result is the mode?

_____

28. Can you determine the mean biopsy result? Why or why not?

_____

29. What is the median type of HPV infection?

_____

30. What is the mode for the type of HPV infection?

_____

31. The study reports the association between the type of HPV infection and cervical cell abnormalities has a *p*-value of 0.06. If the alpha for the study is set at 0.05, what should the researcher conclude regarding the null hypothesis? Why?

_____

32. What is the prevalence of HPV infection in this sample?

_____

33. If instead of an alpha of 0.05 the researchers decided to set this pilot study's alpha at 0.10, what would the researcher conclude about the null hypothesis ($p = 0.06$)?

_____

34. If the researcher rejects the null but does so in error, what type of error could he or she be making? What does this type of error mean?

_____

35. If the researcher does find a statistically significant difference, does this mean it is a clinically significant difference?

_____

36. If the researcher reports an alpha of 0.05 and a *p*-value of 0.09, are the results clinically significant? Why or why not?

_____

37. Write what you would conclude about the null hypothesis with the following results at the two different levels of alpha:

Study	p-Value	Alpha = 0.05	Alpha = 0.10
A	0.0647		
B	0.912		
C	0.1567		
D	0.0211		
E	0.081		

38. Using the table, if the researcher is incorrect about the decision made regarding the null hypothesis, which studies could be a type one error at an alpha of 0.05? Why?

39. Using the table, if the researcher is incorrect about the decision made regarding the null hypothesis, which studies could be a type one error at an alpha of 0.10? Why?

40. Does increasing the alpha increase or decrease the risk of a type one error?

ANSWERS TO CHAPTER 6 REVIEW QUESTIONS

1. H_0: There is no relationship between years worked and salary earned.

   H_1: There is a relationship between years worked and salary earned. Or: More years worked is related to a higher earned salary.

3. Reject the null. The p-value is significant; therefore, you conclude that there is a relationship between years worked and salary earned.

5. You do not know. It depends on the clinical judgment of the experts in clinical care. You may be one of them!

7. Alpha of 0.01

9. Reject the null. There is an association between a positive toxicology screen for Rohypnol and signs of sexual assault.

11. Qualitative

13. $15 \div 45 = 33.3\%$

15. $35 \div 45 = 77.7\%$

17. There is a relationship between the strain of HPV infection and cervical cell abnormalities.

19. Nominal

21. Two-staged cluster sample

23. $62 \div 120 = 52\%$

25. $104 \div 120 = 87\%$

27. CIN I

29. Low risk

31. Fail to reject the null, $p > $ alpha

33. Reject the null, $p < $ alpha

35. No, in addition to being statistically significant, experts in the field must also support the argument that it is a clinically significant difference.

37.

Study	*p*-Value	Alpha $= 0.05$	Alpha $= 0.10$
A	0.0647	Fail to reject the null	Reject the null
B	0.912	Fail to reject the null	Fail to reject the null
C	0.1567	Fail to reject the null	Fail to reject the null
D	0.0211	Reject the null	Reject the null
E	0.081	Fail to reject the null	Reject the null

39. A, D, E—in order to make a type one error you must reject the null incorrectly.

SAMPLE SIZE, EFFECT SIZE, AND POWER

SO HOW MANY SUBJECTS DO I NEED?

By the end of the chapter students will be able to:

- Describe the components of sample size calculation and relate them to one another.

- Recognize a type two error and contrast it with a type one error.

- Estimate the chance of a type two or type one error in a current research article.

- Interpret the power in a current research study and how it would affect the necessary sample size if it were increased or decreased.

- Calculate the anticipated effect size in a study.

KEY TERMS

Alpha (α)
The chance of making a type one error.

Beta (β)
The chance of making a type two error.

Effect size
The extent to which a difference/relationship exists between variables in a population (the size of the difference you are attempting to find).

Power
The ability to find a difference or an association when one actually exists.

Power analysis
How sample sizes are calculated.

Type one error
The error made when a researcher incorrectly rejects the null hypothesis, when he or she concludes there is a significant relationship but there really is not.

Type two error
The error made when a researcher accepts the null incorrectly, missing an association that is really there (sometimes called a power error because the researcher may not have enough power to find an association that really exists).

EFFECT SIZE

You've gotten pretty far in your research. You've noticed clinical associations, examined descriptive data, evaluated the measurement tools, generated a hypothesis, and decided on your sampling method. Now you need to determine how many subjects you will actually need to sample. This decision is largely dependent on the **effect size**, or the size of the difference between group means that exists within the population.

Effect size and sample size are inversely proportional: As one increases, the other decreases. This fact surprises a lot of people, but it is not too difficult to grasp if you think about it. If you are anticipating a large difference (i.e., a strong effect), you may need only a small sample. If you are anticipating a small difference (i.e., a weak effect), you may need to collect a very large sample. The closer the two groups' means are to each other in the population, the more information you need to demonstrate they are different.

One way to determine effect size mathematically is to divide the difference between the mean in the experimental group and the mean in the control group by the standard deviation of the control group. Some statisticians prefer to delineate small, medium, and large effect sizes based on the statistical procedure being conducted whereas others use general guidelines such as those that follow. Let's look at an example.

Grove (2007) prefers to use the following values:

- A weak effect size is < 0.3 (or −0.3).
- A moderate effect size is 0.3–0.5 (or −0.3 to −0.5).
- A strong effect size is > 0.5 (or −0.5).

If you want to know how much of an actual difference in means this is, you can multiply the effect size by the standard deviation in the control group. For example, in a study on the effect of an intervention with premature infants, the control group had a standard deviation of 10 days.

- An intervention with a weak effect size would be associated with a decrease of less than 3 days of prematurity (0.1 or 0.2 × 10).
- A moderate effect size would be associated with a decrease of 3–5 days in prematurity (0.3 to 0.5 × 10).

- A decrease in more than 5 days of prematurity would be a large effect size (0.6 [or more] × 10).

The size of the sample directly relates to the **power** of the study, or the ability to find a difference when one actually exists. The two concepts are directly proportional; that is, as one increases the other must as well. Power is defined as the likelihood of rejecting the null hypothesis correctly; that is, you say there is a relationship and difference, and you are correct. It is usually considered adequate to have a power of 0.80 or 80% (Munro, 2005).

FROM THE STATISTICIAN *Brendan Heavey*

The Four Pillars of Study Planning

Whenever I plan a study, particularly in deciding on sample size, I like to think of myself as juggling four mysterious balls, which represent:

1. Alpha level
2. Effect size
3. Power
4. Sample size

None of these balls is labeled, but knowing any three enables me to know the fourth without seeing any labels.

The **alpha** level is the probability of rejecting H_0 (the null hypothesis) given that it is true. For our present purposes, setting alpha to 0.05 every time is acceptable.

Think of *effect size* as the amount of difference between what was hypothesized in H_0 and what we find in our study. When planning a study, we try to ensure that true differences result in statistical significance, but false differences do not. So the smaller the difference is that we want to detect, the larger the number of cases we need to look at. (Effect size is inversely proportional to sample size.)

How does the researcher decide on the size of the difference to look at? This is not a statistical question; it has to be determined by previous studies or by some other scientific means. This determination can be tricky. Statisticians rely heavily on investigators to provide them with a difference that is clinically important. Determining the degree of difference

(continues)

FROM THE STATISTICIAN *Brendan Heavey*

can be a major undertaking and requires much background research. Sometimes figuring this out takes longer than completing the whole study!

The third concept, power, is probably the most difficult concept to grasp in any introductory statistics class. Many beginning students have trouble understanding it. You can think of power as the probability of rejecting the null hypothesis when the alternative hypothesis is true. Power depends on the truth of the hypothesis under study and totally ignores what happens when the null hypothesis is true. Other analysis methods (specifically, setting an alpha threshold) take into account when the null hypothesis is true. Power takes the analysis a step further.

Most studies typically consider 80% power as adequate; that is, if the alternative hypothesis is true you have a probability of at least 80% that you will reject the null hypothesis. This standard percentage is based on convention, just like having an alpha of 0.05. To increase power (the probability of rejecting the null when the alternative is true) and maintain the same alpha level (the probability of incorrectly rejecting the null), you need to increase the sample size. In simpler terms, increasing power requires increasing sample size in order to maintain the same alpha level. Power is *directly* proportional to sample size: When sample size increases, power increases. If you want to increase power, increase your sample size.

Sample size (represented as *n*) is the fourth ball juggled in study planning. Statisticians always, always, always want to increase sample size. Increasing sample size is rarely a bad thing. The problem is that increasing sample size usually means increasing the cost of a study, so statisticians use other approaches to decide on an acceptable sample size.

There are two usual ways of planning a study. The first involves defining the desired effect size and then figuring out the sample size needed to achieve the related power. Statisticians usually choose 0.80 or 80% power and then decide whether the study is possible given the required sample size. In other words, the juggler in me:

- Selects alpha (juggled object 1) as 0.05.
- Defines the effect size of interest (juggled object 2).
- Sets power to 80% (juggled object 3).
- This leaves me with one last juggling object, the sample size, which is completely determined by the other three. The equations you will use to make these determinations are determined by the statistical technique you will employ in your study.

I then do a cost/benefit analysis on my final sample size to determine whether the study should be done. For example, if the cost of acquiring the necessary data for an adequately sized sample is $100,000, the researcher has to determine whether the benefit associated with the anticipated results will have a value greater than this investment.

Another approach to study planning is to determine what sample size is available and then what effect size is needed to achieve the appropriate power level (again, usually 0.80 or 80%). In this case, alpha is again set to 0.05, sample size is set to our determined limit, and power is set to 0.80 or 80%. That leaves the juggled object of effect size to be figured out, and it can now be determined based on the other three. Finally, the researcher must determine whether the effect size is interesting enough to warrant performing the study (this usually involves a cost/benefit analysis).

(continues)

FROM THE STATISTICIAN *Brendan Heavey*

For instance, oversupplementation of vitamin A has been shown to cause liver damage. We design a study to determine whether the damage is caused by reduced blood flow to the liver. We have been given a National Institutes of Health award for outstanding merit in clinical research based on our previous work with EpiPens. The award is for $500,000 and must be put toward further research. With this amount, we can enroll 25 subjects in our study ($n = 25$), who will be asked to come to the hospital for 4 hours, fill out a survey, have blood drawn, and undergo a positron emission tomography (PET) scan. We set the alpha level at 0.05 and power at 0.8 or 80% which we figure will be sufficient to predict an increase of 0.8 mL/min/g of blood flow or higher. Unfortunately, with this size sample, we can detect only a very large difference (i.e., effect size) in blood flow to the liver. By the time patients have that much difference in blood flow to the liver, they will have already exhibited other detectable signs and symptoms of liver disease, so the effect size we could find with this sample size is too large to be clinically useful. We need to be able to find a smaller difference for the results to be clinically useful; specifically, the study would be useful only if we can predict a difference of 0.08 mL/min/g or lower. Detecting this small an effect size requires us to enroll more subjects than we can afford with this grant money. Can you figure out what other factors we might adjust to make this study feasible?

That's the juggling act. These four concepts are all interrelated. Changing one can affect all three of the others. Note that alpha is rarely changed to accommodate lack of funding. Instead, we first reduce power because in the scientific community it is generally worse to give up on answers that might be right than it is to waste time on answers that are probably wrong. We'll look at this reasoning more in depth in the next "From the Statistician."

TYPE TWO ERROR

Any time you make a decision, there is a chance that you will make a mistake (like ordering garlic sushi on a blind date—big mistake!). When your decision involves failing to reject the null hypothesis, you must consider the possibility of a **type two error**, that is, the error made when you fail to reject the null *incorrectly*, missing an association that is really there. These errors usually occur because the sample wasn't large enough and the study therefore didn't have enough power to find a difference that really existed. Hence type two errors are also frequently called power errors.

Any hypothesis test has the risk of committing a type two error. This risk is represented by **beta (β)**. You can calculate your chance of a type two error fairly simply. Given that there really is a relationship or difference between the variables you are examining, you will either correctly identify it (i.e., reject H_0 correctly = power) or you will incorrectly miss it (type two error). Because there is a 100% chance that you will be *either* correct *or* incorrect (pretty much true for all life decisions), you know that:

Power (correctly rejecting H_0) + Beta (chance of making a type two error) = 100%

Therefore, if there is an 80% chance that you are correct and find the relationship (power), the chance of a type two error is 20%.

On a practical basis, the convention is to set beta at 20%. So you can quickly calculate beta by subtracting the power of the study (usually 80%, or 0.80) from one: $1 - 0.80 = 0.20$.

A QUICK REVIEW OF TYPE ONE AND TYPE TWO ERRORS

Type one and type two errors seem relatively straightforward until you start trying to think about the both of them together. Sort them out like this. The life decisions rule is that, no matter what you are deciding, there are usually two outcomes: You are (1) correct or (2) incorrect. (All of the philosopher-students are horrified that I see things this way, but bear with me.) The question that all research studies ask is whether the null hypothesis is true: The two variables have no relationship, difference, or association between them. In actuality it may be true or it may not be true, and you can reject or fail to reject the null hypothesis in either of these situations.

If the null hypothesis *really is true* and there is no relationship or difference between the variables, you can conclude one of two things:

- You can fail to reject it. You are *correct* in this situation and the probability of reaching this conclusion is 1—alpha (usually 0.05) or 95%.
- Or you can reject it. Then you are incorrect and are making a **type one error**. The probability of reaching this conclusion is equal to alpha, usually 5%.

If the null hypothesis is really not true and there is a relationship between the variables, you can conclude one of two things:

- You can fail to reject it. In this case, you are *incorrect* and are making a type two error. The probability of doing so is equal to β (usually 0.20 or 20%).
- Or you can reject it *correctly*. The probability of reaching this conclusion is $1 - \beta$ (usually 80%), which is also the power of your study.

Getting the two types of errors confused is easy, so thinking of them in terms of the null hypothesis is helpful. If you reject the null *and are incorrect* you are making a type one error. If you fail to reject the null *and are incorrect* you are making a type two error. Of course, if you are already a statistician, you may not need this tip—but the rest of us do get confused sometimes!

SAMPLE SIZE

All these ideas are related in that you need to understand them to determine your sample size. Before you even begin a study, you need to decide how many subjects to sample. That decision depends on the size of the difference you are looking to detect. In other words, the sample size you need should give you adequate power to correctly reject the null hypothesis. **Power analysis** is how sample sizes are calculated. The many different equations for calculating sample sizes depend on the statistical techniques the study utilizes. Luckily for you, these calculations are beyond the scope of this text. (So you have something to look forward to in your next stats class!) However, power analysis involves some central concepts no

FROM THE STATISTICIAN   *Brendan Heavey*

Which Error Is Worse? The Lesser of Two Evils

How do we decide how many subjects to enroll for a study? This is a bread-and-butter question for statisticians, and their answer involves a concept that many people don't understand. Often statisticians have to decide whether it is worse to commit a type one error or a type two error. Statisticians can debate the question for hours, but in this country's legal system—as well as in most of the world's scientific community and real-life situations—committing a type one error is definitely worse.

Let me explain that point. In any court case, four different scenarios are possible, just as in the hypothesis test explanation. See **Figure 7-1**. The U.S. legal system is based on the principle that people are innocent until proven guilty (H_0: The defendant is not guilty). Inherent in that principle is a subprinciple that sending an innocent person to jail is much worse than letting a guilty person walk. This is the reason for such an enormous appeals process and why you cannot be tried twice for the same offense.

In statistics we have a similar philosophy:

- We put a hard cap on alpha (the probability of a false positive) of about 0.05.
- We shoot for a power of about 80%.
- So beta, the probability of a false negative, is set around 0.20 (a much more likely outcome than the accepted probability for a false positive).

We do the same thing in statistics that the U.S. court system does; we just charge less per hour than the average lawyer! Medical researchers play by much the same rules. Often, researchers find sets of genes that they think may be involved in causing cancer or some other debilitating disease. Once they have found a set of interest, the next step is to test all of them simultaneously in groups of control versus cancerous subjects. This research process can involve upward of 50,000 genes in thousands of subjects at once. What would go through your head if you had to decide how to run this large and complex analysis? You would have to sort each gene into one of the four categories from the 2×2 table. Most of the genes would have the same expression in both cancerous and control tissue, and you could eliminate them from contention. Beyond that set, you'd have to decide which is worse: rejecting the one lone gene that may be the cause of cancer *or* wasting time sifting through too many genes that don't have anything to do with your analysis question. Obviously, rejecting the right answer is the worse of the two evils. Unfortunately, this means that scientists' time gets wasted all too often!

matter which calculation you are using. The sample size you need in your study depends on the following:

- *Effect size:* The anticipated difference you expect to see

- *How much type one error you can tolerate:* Alpha, or chances of incorrectly saying there is a difference
- *Power:* The ability to detect a difference that really exists

FIGURE 7-1	**Criminal Status and Trial Results.**

		Truth	
		Defendant is innocent.	**Defendant is guilty.**
Result of the Trial	Defendant is convicted.	Major problem TYPE ONE ERROR	No problem $1 - \beta$ = power
	Defendant is acquitted.	No problem $1 -$ alpha	Minor problem TYPE TWO ERROR

Even after calculating the necessary sample size, you may need to increase it if you anticipate a large number of dropouts or a high nonresponse rate. For example, many nurses who are asked about their sexual orientation may choose not to respond to that question, leaving you with too small of a sample size to draw any conclusions. Likewise, if you are conducting a study over a long period of time, a number of participants will be lost to follow-up or will be unable to participate for various reasons, such as death, illness, relocation, and the like. These factors all need to be considered when calculating the number of subjects to include in a sample.

When a sample size is too small, you have a greater chance of a type two error. If you don't have enough subjects, you may not find a statistical difference even though one exists. However, when the sample is too large, you not only waste time and money, but also have a greater chance of a type one error.

You might find a statistical difference that really isn't there and promote a treatment or course of action that may not be the best option for patients.

SUMMARY

Way to go! You have completed the chapter. Now for a quick review.

- The effect size is the extent to which a difference/relationship exists between the variables under study in the population. It is also the size or difference you are attempting to find in your study.
- The power of the study is the ability to find a difference when one actually does exist.
- A power analysis is how sample sizes are actually calculated.
- A type one error is when you reject the null hypothesis and are incorrect. In other words, you stated that there was

a difference in the variable when there really was not.

- A type two error is when you fail to reject the null incorrectly, meaning you miss a relationship that does exist.

- Beta is another name for the chance of committing a type two error.
- The sample size you need in your study depends on the effect size or the anticipated difference you expect to see.

CHAPTER 7 REVIEW QUESTIONS

Questions 1–14: You are asked to develop a study for a pharmaceutical company to determine whether taking one tablet of drug A is related to lower total cholesterol levels.

1. What is your independent variable?

_____

2. What is your dependent variable?

_____

3. How could you measure your dependent variable quantitatively?

_____

   a. Would this be a continuous or categorical variable?

_____

   b. What level of measurement would this variable be?

_____

4. How could you measure your dependent variable qualitatively?

_____

_____

   a. Would this be a continuous or categorical variable?

_____

   b. What level of measurement would this variable be?

_____

5. You chose to measure taking one tablet of drug A as a yes/no question.

_____

   a. What level of measurement is this variable?

_____

   b. What would be the best measure of central tendency?

_____

6. Write a null hypothesis for your study.

7. Write an alternative hypothesis for your study.

8. If you select an alpha of 0.05 and a power of 80%, what does your decision mean?

9. Your study has an alpha of 0.05. Your statistical test determines that the p-value for the relationship between taking one tablet of drug A daily and lowering cholesterol is 0.02. What do you conclude?

10. If your conclusion was actually a type one error, what do you know about taking drug A and cholesterol levels?

11. Based on the preliminary pilot study you conducted, the drug company decides to fund a large-scale clinical trial. This trial results in a p-value of 0.07. What is your conclusion?

12. You determine after the trial that the actual effect size from the medication was smaller than you initially thought. Knowing this, you conclude you may have made what type of error in your conclusion?

13. What was the most likely cause of this error?

14. If your study had an alpha of 0.05 and a power of 80%, calculate the chance that you made a type two error.

15. In each of the following instances, identify which type of error is potentially being made: type one or type two.

    a. Your study concludes that ambulation post-op day 1 from hip replacement surgery is associated with shorter hospital stays.

    b. Your study examining the relationship between head trauma and grand mal seizures has an alpha of 0.10 and a beta of 0.80. Your statistical analysis reports a p-value of 0.06.

    c. Your study finds no relationship between vitamin E consumption and skin cancer.

    d. Your original intention was to enroll 500 subjects in your study, but only 256 completed both a pre- and posttest. You are concerned about what type of error?

    e. Your study has an alpha of 0.05 and a beta of 0.90. You examine a sample of circus workers to determine whether they have higher levels of lung cancer. Your statistical analysis finds a p-value of 0.04.

    f. The poorly designed pilot study examining the relationship between mold exposure and asthma reports a small effect size. You recruit a large sample to attempt to enable your research team to successfully detect this effect size. Having a larger sample size increases the risk of making what type of error?

16. You have two samples of adults preparing for barium enema tests the next day. The control group consumes 2 oz of milk of magnesia with a mean average of 120 ml and a standard deviation of 10 ml of water. The second group is advised to consume more water with their milk of magnesia, and they average 124 ml with a standard deviation of 12 ml of water. Calculate the effect size in this experiment. Is it small, moderate, or large by Grove's standards?

Questions 17–30: A study anticipates subjects treated with drug A will have substantial improvement in their neuropathy symptoms.

17. If the study measures treatment with drug A as given or not given, what level of measurement is this variable?

18. If the study measures treatment with drug A as not given, low dose, or high dose, what level of measurement is this variable?

19. If the study measures treatment with drug A as 0 mg/day, 100 mg/day, or 200 mg/day, what level of measurement is this variable?

20. If the study measures neuropathy symptoms as present or not present, what level of measurement is this variable?

21. If the study measures neuropathy symptoms on a scale of 1 10, what level of measurement is this variable?

22. If the study measures neuropathy symptoms as mild, moderate, or severe, what level of measurement is this variable?

_____

23. The study anticipates subjects treated with drug A will have substantial improvement in their neuropathy symptoms. What effect size is anticipated, and what does that mean in terms of the sample size needed?

_____

24. The researcher knows of a validated survey instrument to measure neuropathy symptoms, but it has 500 questions and requires a college-level reading ability to understand. These features limit what aspect of the measurement tool?

_____

25. The 10-question survey instrument used to measure neuropathy symptoms in this study was compared to a previously validated 500-question version and similar results were obtained. This is an example of establishing what type of validity?

_____

26. This large-scale trial will have measurements collected by 14 data collectors at three sites. Discuss an aspect of reliability that will be critical to assess to avoid compromising the validity of the study.

_____

27. The neuropathy survey has a 96% sensitivity. What does this mean?

_____

28. This study, which examines treating patients with drug A and neuropathy symptoms, utilizes an alpha of 0.05 and reports a p-value of 0.30. What should the researcher decide about the null hypothesis? Why?

_____

29. If this decision about the null hypothesis is incorrect, what type of error could it be?

_____

30. In the following table, fill in the researcher's decision about the null hypothesis at the indicated alpha level as well as what potential error it could be if this decision is incorrect.

p-Value	Alpha Value	Null Hypothesis Decision	Potential Error
0.061	0.05		
0.101	0.05		
0.022	0.05		
0.167	0.10		
0.014	0.10		
0.079	0.05		
0.079	0.10		

ANSWERS TO CHAPTER 7 REVIEW QUESTIONS

1. Drug A

3. Serum cholesterol, (a) continuous, (b) interval/ratio

5. (a) nominal, (b) mode

7. Answers may vary. Example: Taking drug A is associated with a change in cholesterol level. Or: Drug A lowers cholesterol level.

9. Reject the null hypothesis. There is a relationship between taking drug A and cholesterol levels.

11. Fail to reject the null; there is not enough evidence to show a relationship between drug A and cholesterol levels.

13. Inadequate power due to too small of a sample to detect this effect size

15. a. Reject the null, may be a type one error.
    b. Reject the null, may be a type one error.
    c. Fail to reject the null, may be a type two error.

    d. Fail to reject the null, may be a type two error due to inadequate sample.
    e. Reject the null, may be a type one error.
    f. Reject the null, may be a type one error.

17. Nominal

19. Ratio

21. Interval

23. Large effect size is anticipated, so only a small sample should be necessary to detect it on a statistically significant level.

25. Convergent validity

27. If the patient has neuropathy there is a 96% chance that the survey will indicate this result.

29. Type two

CHAPTER 8

CHI-SQUARE

IS THERE A DIFFERENCE?

OBJECTIVES

By the end of the chapter students will be able to:

- Identify conditions under which the chi-square test is appropriate.
- Identify the question the chi-square test is designed to answer.
- Formulate a null and an alternative hypothesis.
- Formulate a 2×2 table from an existing data set.
- Interpret an SPSS printout of a chi-square test, determine what action to take with regard to the null hypothesis, and justify this decision in statistically correct terminology.

- Identify a current research article that uses a chi-square test, determine the level of measurement of the variables used and whether the results are statistically significant, and utilize this information to draw a statistical conclusion.
- Debate whether clinical recommendations should be made from a research article's conclusion, and prepare a public health report using this information.

KEY TERMS

Chi-square (X^2)
A test used with independent samples of nominal- or ordinal-level data.

Degrees of freedom (*df*)
The number values that are "free to be unknown."

Null hypothesis
Means that there is no relationship/association or difference between or amongst the variables of interest.

CHI-SQUARE (X^2) TEST

Recall that, in most experiments, the **null hypothesis** is that there is no relationship/association or difference between the study groups or samples. So how can we test to see whether there really is no difference? That's what we will discuss here: an actual test to see whether there is a statistically significant difference.

In this chapter, we are going to talk about the **chi-square (X^2) test**, which is appropriate when you are working with independent samples and an outcome or dependent variable that is nominal- or ordinal-level data. You already know that nominal-level data tells you that there is a difference in the quality of a variable, whereas ordinal-level data has a rank order so that one level is greater than or less than another.

For example, suppose you are an operating room nurse and you want to see whether there is a difference between male and female postoperative patients in the need for a postoperative transfusion. Gender is the variable that identifies your sample groups. You want to compare a sample of men and a sample of women. Your outcome or dependent variable is postoperative transfusion, which is measured at a nominal level (yes/no). Now

you want to see whether the frequencies you observe are different from the frequencies you would expect if the variables were independent or not related.

THE NULL AND ALTERNATIVE HYPOTHESES

So let's formulate a null hypothesis and an alternative hypothesis using the standard notation, which looks like this:

H_0: This is how statisticians indicate the null hypothesis.
H_1: This notation indicates the alternative hypothesis.

Here are our hypotheses:

H_0: There is no difference in the need for a postoperative transfusion among men and women.
H_1: The need for a postoperative transfusion is different for men and women.

2 × 2 TABLE

Your next step is to set up another 2 × 2 table. Statisticians love these! See **Figure 8-1**.

FIGURE 8-1	**Gender and Postoperative Transfusion Status.**

	Male	**Female**	**Total**
Transfused	20 (A)	30 (B)	50 (A + B)
Not transfused	30 (C)	20 (D)	50 (C + D)
Total	50 (A + C)	50 (B + D)	100 (A + B + C + D)

DEGREES OF FREEDOM

Before you determine statistical significance you will need to determine the **degrees of freedom (*df*)**, which is the number values that are "free to be unknown" once the row and column totals are in a 2 × 2 contingency table. With a chi-square test, the degrees of freedom are equal to the number of rows minus one times the number of columns minus one:

$$df = (2-1) \times (2-1)$$
$$df = 1 \times 1 = 1$$

All 2 × 2 tables have one degree of freedom. In other words, once you know the row and column totals and one other cell value in the table, you can figure out all the rest of the cell values in the table and they do not change unless the original cell value changes. This is why there is only one value that is "free to be unknown."

STATISTICAL SIGNIFICANCE

Once you put your data into a statistical program, it will compute the expected values for each of these cells, assuming the two variables are independent. You will then need to apply the chi-square test to see whether the observed values are significantly different from the expected values at one degree of freedom.

- If the X^2 result has a *p*-value that is significant (usually < 0.05 depending on the alpha you use), then you reject the null hypothesis that the two variables are independent and conclude that there is an association between gender and postoperative transfusion. Postoperative transfusion rates are significantly different for men and women.

- If the X^2 value is greater than the alpha you selected (e.g., if your alpha is 0.05 and the *p*-value is 0.09), then the result is not statistically significant and you fail to reject the null hypothesis. Your study does not have the statistical strength for you to say the variables are not related. In this case you conclude that postoperative transfusion rates are not significantly different for men and women. Remember that this may be because there really isn't a difference in postoperative transfusion rates for men and women or because of other reasons, such as your sample size was too small.

DIRECTION OF THE RELATIONSHIP

Also note that the chi-square test doesn't tell you the direction of the relationship or difference. If the p-value for your X^2 is significant, all you know is that you can reject the null and that there is a statistically significant difference in your outcome variable between the two samples. As the statistical wizard that you are, you then look again at your data to determine what that difference is. For example, if you had a statistically significant X^2 in the example about gender and postoperative transfusions, you could go back and look at which gender had more transfusions. In this sample, a larger portion of the women needed transfusions. Given your statistically significant result, you could conclude that, for this sample, women are more likely to need a postoperative transfusion than men.

FROM THE STATISTICIAN *Brendan Heavey*

Pearson's Chi-Square Test for Association

The chi-square test is one of the simplest tests available in a subset of statistics called categorical data analysis. The majority of theories relating to categorical data analysis started to be developed around the turn of the 20th century. Karl Pearson (1857–1936) was a very important statistician from England who is responsible for first developing the chi-squared distribution. Pearson was an arrogant man who frequently butted heads with colleagues. He specifically argued the intelligence and merits of a young statistician named R.A. Fisher (1890–1962), who has since become established as one of the most important scientists of all time. The two men argued over many different things. Fisher was concerned about what would happen to Pearson's chi-squared statistic when sample sizes were extremely low, and Pearson didn't think it was a problem.

Fisher contributed a number of fundamentals of statistical science, but specifically in introductory categorical data analysis he developed the Fisher exact test. This test is now commonly used in place of Pearson's chi-square test when the sample size of any cell in the data is less than 5 (because, in the end, Fisher's arguments with Pearson proved correct). Fisher also used properties derived from Pearson's chi-squared distribution to show that Gregor Mendel, the eminent geneticist and Augustinian priest who theorized about the inheritance of genetic traits using peas, most likely derived many of his theories based on fabricated data. (Fisher remained convinced that one of Mendel's assistants was responsible for the fabrication; Mendel is still considered a very gifted geneticist.) In any event, the two tests—Pearson's chi-square test and Fisher's exact test—are now very common statistics to use in clinical trials and scientific research. Specifically, their use is very popular when a researcher wants to test whether a new treatment or therapy is better than the so-called gold standard already in use.

The null hypothesis that is tested in both these tests is:

H_0: The proportions being compared are equal in the population.

(continues)

FROM THE STATISTICIAN *Brendan Heavey*

Here is a motivating example, one that's slightly more difficult than the one in the main text. This time we'll use a variable that has more than just two categories.

Suppose we want to study the effect of a husband's occupation on a woman's marital happiness in a clinically relevant population. Our null hypothesis is:

H_0: Husband's occupation has no effect on women's marital happiness in this subset of occupations in the population we have sampled from.

To conduct the study, we enroll 1,868 women and ask them to rate the happiness of their marriage on the following four-point scale:

1. Very happy
2. Pretty happy
3. Happy
4. Not too happy

The results are shown in **Figure 8-2**. Now, if you plug these values into any statistical program (or use the From the Statistician: Methods section from this chapter to hand-calculate the values), you'll see that the p-value for the difference between the happiness of the wives of statisticians versus those of male supermodels is so low that it is estimated at 0. Now you know that there is an association between the husband's occupation and the wife's marital happiness (because

FIGURE 8-2 **Husbands' Occupation and Wives' Report of Marital Happiness.**

Marital Happiness	Husbands' Occupation		Total
	Statistician	Male Supermodel	
Very happy	800	25	825
Pretty happy	706	10	716
Happy	200	25	225
Not too happy	2	100	102
Total	1708	160	1868

(continues)

your *p*-value is less than alpha, meaning it is significant). So you reject the null hypothesis that there isn't a relationship between husband's occupation and a wife's marital happiness.

But what else might you like to know? Let's say that a friend is dating a statistician and a male supermodel and that they both intend to propose this evening. What advice would you give your friend? Which might be the better choice to ensure long-term marital satisfaction? Remember that the chi-square test tells you only that there is a better choice, not which one it is. But you remember from your college stats class that you can determine which is better by looking at the data. The proportion of wives married to statisticians who reported being happy or higher was 99.9% (1,706 ÷ 1,708), whereas the proportion of wives married to supermodels who reported being happy or higher was 37.5% (60 ÷ 160). So, assuming your friend wants to get married in the first place, which proposal should she accept? (*Hint:* In the statistics books, the statisticians always live happily ever after!)

Here are three health-related studies that all demonstrate the use of this statistic:

1. Corless et al. (2009) examined the effect of marijuana use versus over-the-counter medications for the relief of symptoms and side effects associated with HIV medication.
2. Tobian et al. (2009) investigated the contribution of different variables to determine whether circumcision was an effective strategy for syphilis prevention in a community in Uganda.
3. Anifantaki (2009) examined the relationship between daily interruption of sedative infusions and the duration of mechanical ventilation required in patients in an adult surgical intensive care unit.

(**Note:** All the anecdotal information regarding Spearman and Fisher came from Agresti's (2002) landmark book on the subject, *Categorical Data Analysis*.)

WHEN *NOT* TO USE CHI-SQUARE: ASSUMPTIONS AND SPECIAL CASES

In a few situations, you might be inclined to use a chi-square test because you have an outcome or dependent variable at the nominal level, but the test wouldn't be a good choice. The chi-square test includes some additional assumptions (in addition to requiring a nominal-level outcome or dependent variable), which must be met for the test to be used appropriately.

All cells within the 2 × 2 table must have an observed value greater than or equal to 5. If at least one cell in your 2 × 2 table has an observed value less than 5 you should use the Fisher exact test *instead. You should also note that if any of the cells in the frequency table has greater than 5 but fewer than 10 expected observations, you can still use the chi-square test but you need to do a Yates continuity correction as well.* The really nice thing in this day and age is that many statistical programs automatically make this correction when this condition occurs, saving you the time and trouble of doing it manually. You might want to look for it on your next SPSS printout.

The sample should be random and independent. Here's an example of a violation of this assumption: Your study involved measuring the need for postoperative transfusion among husbands and wives who underwent a particular procedure. (Because these subjects are related to each other they are not independent—once you included the wife in the study, the husband was included as well,

so his participation was "dependent" on his wife being selected to participate.) In this case, the sample is not independent and random. Instead, the sample is now matched, or paired, and a test called the McNemar test is the correct choice to use for the analysis.

(Both the Fisher and the McNemar tests are based on the same idea as the chi-square, but they have mathematical adjustments to accommodate the violation in the assumptions of the chi-square test.)

FROM THE STATISTICIAN *Brendan Heavey*

Methods: Calculating Pearson's Chi-Square Test by Hand

Figure 8-3 is a repeat of **Figure 8-2**, for easier reference.

1. The first step is to calculate the expected frequency from each cell with the following formula:

$$\text{Expected frequency} = \frac{\text{Row total} \times \text{Column total}}{\text{Grand total}}$$

FIGURE 8-3 **Husbands' Occupation and Wives' Report of Marital Happiness.**

Marital Happiness	Husbands' Occupation		
	Statistician	Male Supermodel	Total
Very happy	800	25	825
Pretty happy	706	10	716
Happy	200	25	225
Not too happy	2	100	102
Total	1708	160	1868

(continues)

FROM THE STATISTICIAN *Brendan Heavey*

The results are shown in **Figure 8-4**.

FIGURE 8-4 **Expected Frequencies for Husbands' Occupation and Wives' Marital Satisfaction.**

Expected Frequencies

	Statistician	Male Supermodel
Very happy	$(825 \times 1708) \div 1868 = 754.334$	$(825 \times 160) \div 1868 = 70.66$
Pretty happy	$(716 \times 1708) \div 1868 = 654.67$	$(716 \times 160) \div 1868 = 61.33$
Happy	$(225 \times 1708) \div 1868 = 205.73$	$(225 \times 160) \div 1868 = 19.27$
Not too happy	$(102 \times 1708) \div 1868 = 93.26$	$(102 \times 160) \div 1868 = 8.734$

2. Now compute the statistic:

$$\sum \frac{(\text{Observed} - \text{Expected})^2}{\text{Expected}}$$

The big sigma (Σ) character just means to sum everything over all the cells; in our case we calculate:

$$\frac{(800 - 754.34)^2}{754.37} + \frac{(706 - 654.67)^2}{654.67} + \frac{(200 - 205.73)^2}{205.73} + \frac{(2 - 93.26)^2}{93.26}$$

$$+ \frac{(25 - 70.66)^2}{70.66} + \frac{(10 - 61.33)^2}{61.33} + \frac{(25 - 19.27)^2}{19.27} + \frac{(100 - 8.74)^2}{8.74}$$

which results in 1123.8.

3. We then apply the formula for calculating the degrees of freedom for a chi-square test:

$$(\text{Number of rows} - 1)(\text{Number of columns} - 1)$$

In this case, the degrees of freedom is:

$$3 \times 1 = 3$$

4. We can then look up the *p*-value for this test statistic from a table of the chi-square distribution with degrees of freedom:

$p < 0.0001$.

SUMMARY

There are two main points to review in this chapter. First, you should understand the concept of the null hypothesis. The null hypothesis is that there is no relationship/association or difference between the variables of interest. Second, the chi-square test is used to look for a statistically significant difference or relationship when you have a nominal- or ordinal-level dependent or outcome variable.

- If the chi-square test result has a *p-value* that is significant (less than 0.05 or whatever alpha you use), then you reject the null hypothesis.
- If the chi-square test result is not statistically significant (greater than 0.05 or the alpha of choice), then you fail to reject the null hypothesis.

The chi-square test does not tell you the direction of the relationship; only you can make that interpretation.

That about wraps up this chapter. Not too bad, right?

CHAPTER 8 REVIEW QUESTIONS

Questions 1–11: A study is completed to examine the relationship between gender and sports participation. It is conducted by randomly surveying ninth graders at Smith High School. The collected data is shown in **Figure 8-5**.

1. What level of measurement is gender? Is it continuous or categorical?

_____

_____

2. What level of measurement is sports participation? Is it qualitative or quantitative?

_____

_____

FIGURE 8-5 **Gender and Sports Participation Among Ninth-Grade Students.**

	Male	Female	Total
No sports	30	50	80
Sports participation	70	50	120
Total	100	100	200

3. What measure of central tendency can you determine for sports participation? What is the measure of central tendency for males only? Is the measure of central tendency different for the whole sample?

     _____

     _____

4. If the whole school has 800 students and the ninth grade has 250 students, what percentage of the ninth-grade population did you sample?

     _____

     _____

5. Write an appropriate null hypothesis for this study.

     _____

     _____

6. Write two alternative hypotheses that correspond to your null hypothesis.

     _____

     _____

7. Calculate the chi-square from the 2×2 table in Figure 8-5. The p-value is < 0.005. Is sports participation significantly different for males and females in this sample? (See the From the Statistician: Methods calculation.)

     _____

     _____

8. What should you conclude about your null hypothesis?

     _____

     _____

9. What type of error might you be making?

     _____

     _____

10. If you wanted to make the chance of this type of error smaller, what could you do?

     _____

     _____

11. Why is the chi-square test appropriate for this study?

     _____

     _____

Questions 12–14: After the school instituted a new aerobics program, data was gathered in a follow-up survey administered in all the grades. The collected information is shown in **Figure 8-6**.

12. If the entire school has a population of 800, what percentage of the students are included in your sample?

     _____

     _____

FIGURE 8-6 **Gender and Sports Participation After New Aerobics Program.**

	Male	Female	Total
No sports	60	20	80
Sports participation	140	180	320
Total	200	200	400

Chi-square $= 25$, $p < 0.0001$

13. Is gender related to sports participation in this follow-up survey? If so, which gender is more likely to participate? How many degrees of freedom do you have?

_____

_____

14. Imagine you are the editor of the journal in which an article was submitted for review using a chi-square test to determine whether boys or girls were more likely to participate in sports. After reading it, you realize that the male and female subjects were recruited as brother and sister pairs. What would you conclude about the analysis?

_____

_____

15. You are working in a school-based health center and have developed a new screening tool for suicide risk among adolescent athletes. The pilot of your new screening tool reports female athletes are more likely to attempt suicide when compared to male athletes. These results agree with other published reports from the general adolescent population. This helps establish what type of validity for your new screen?

_____

_____

16. You administer your new screen in your health clinic but find the results confusing. After reviewing your tool, you realize that a mistake was made. When the survey was administered to three of the male sports teams, it was printed on only one side of the paper and should have been copied onto both sides. As a result, half of the survey was missing when it was administered to these three teams. Is your screen reliable? What does this tell you about the validity of the screen in this situation?

_____

_____

17. You correct the copying problem and readminister the screen at another school. After 1 year of follow-up, you get the results shown in **Figure 8-7**. Explain what each box means in plain English.

_____

_____

FIGURE 8-7	Suicide Risk and Screening Results.

	Attempted Suicide	No Suicide Attempt	Total
Screen positive	20	5	25
Screen negative	10	215	225
Total	30	220	250

18. What is the sensitivity of your screen? What does this mean in plain English?

_____

_____

19. What is the specificity of your screen? What does this mean in plain English?

_____

_____

20. What is the positive predictive value (PPV) of your screen? What does this mean in plain English?

_____

_____

21. What is the negative predictive value (NPV) of your screen? What does this mean in plain English?

_____

_____

22. What is the prevalence of suicide attempts in this sample?

_____

_____

FROM THE STATISTICIAN REVIEW QUESTION

23. Would you do the analysis differently if no women were happily married to male supermodels in the From the Statistician section in this chapter?

_____

_____

Questions 24–33: In a random sample of 100 patients with biopsy-confirmed breast cancer, a study examines cancer detection rates with 50 previously collected two-dimensional (2D) mammograms compared to detection rates in 50 previously collected three-dimensional (3D) mammograms. The alpha selected for this pilot study is 0.10 and the power is 0.80.

24. Write a null and alternative hypothesis for this study.

25. What is the independent variable? What level of measurement is it?

26. What is the dependent variable?

27. If cancer detection is measured as yes/no, what level of measurement is this variable?

28. The pilot study reports a chi-square of 2.46. Is there a significant difference between cancer detection rates with these two screening mechanisms?

29. The study reports 2D mammograms detected 70% of cancers and 3D mammograms detected 90% of cancers with a $p = 0.12$. What decision should the researcher make about the null hypothesis?

30. In a larger study with the same parameters, 2D mammograms detected 75% of cancers and 3D mammograms detected 91% of cancers with a $p = 0.01$. What decision should the researcher make about the null hypothesis?

31. Knowing the results of the larger study would make the researcher wonder if the conclusion of the smaller pilot study was what type of error?

32. Additional studies show the sensitivity of the 3D mammogram is 94% and the PPV is 98%. You have a patient with a positive 3D mammogram indicating a high risk of cancer. She wants to know what the chances are that she actually has cancer. What can you tell her?

33. If instead the study design involved looking at 100 women who had both a 2D and a 3D mammogram to determine which screen had higher detection rates, would a chi-square test be appropriate? Why or why not?

Questions 34–39: In a random sample of patients with oropharyngeal cancer, the researcher wishes to determine if there is a relationship between gender and the type of oropharyngeal cancer. The study has an alpha of 0.05 and finds a $p = 0.01$.

34. What is the dependent variable?

_____

_____

35. If the type of oropharyngeal cancer is recorded as oral cavity/pharynx, tongue, mouth, pharynx, and other, what level of measurement is this variable?

_____

_____

36. What would be an appropriate test to use to test the null hypothesis, and why?

_____

_____

37. What decision should be made about the null hypothesis, and why?

_____

_____

38. If this decision is not correct, what potential error could it be?

_____

_____

39. The presence of leukoplakia or erythoplakia in the oropharynx for more than 2 weeks is associated with oropharyngeal cancer. A new tool is developed to screen for oropharyngeal cancer in patients with these symptoms that has an NPV of 84%. Your patient's screen is negative and he wants to know what this means. Explain his result in plain language.

_____

_____

ANSWERS TO CHAPTER 8 REVIEW QUESTIONS

1. Nominal, categorical

3. Nominal, mode, mode = participating in sports for males and for the total sample

5. H_0: There is no relationship between gender and sports participation

7. See **Figure 8-8**.

<table>
<tr><td>FIGURE 8-8</td><td colspan="2">Expected Values for Gender and Sports Participation.</td></tr>
</table>

	Male	**Female**
No sports	$(80 \times 100) \div 200 = 40$	$(80 \times 100) \div 200 = 40$
Sports participation	$(120 \times 100) \div 200 = 60$	$(120 \times 100) \div 200 = 60$

If your alpha is 0.05, then yes, sports participation is significantly different for males and females. This conclusion is because p is significant.

$$\sum \frac{(\text{Observed} - \text{Expected})^2}{\text{Expected}}$$

$$\frac{(30-40)^2}{40} + \frac{(50-40)^2}{40} + \frac{(70-60)^2}{60} + \frac{(50-60)^2}{60}$$

$$= 100/40 + 100/40 + 100/60 + 100/60 = 8.34$$

$$df = 1$$

9. Type one

11. The outcome variable is nominal/ordinal. It is an independent sample and the cell values are all > 5.

13. Yes, females are more likely.

    $df = (\text{Number of rows} - 1) \times (\text{Number of columns} - 1)$
    $= 1 \times 1 = 1$

15. Convergent

17. $20 =$ true positives, $5 =$ false positives, $10 =$ false negatives, $215 =$ true negatives

19. $215/220 = 98\%$. If the subject does not have the disease there is a 98% chance the screen will be negative. A specific screen is good at identifying those without the disease.

21. $215/225 = 96\%$. If the screening test is negative, it is probable that the subject does not have the disease.

ANSWER TO CHAPTER 8 FROM THE STATISTICAN QUESTIONS

23. You would need to use Fisher's exact test because of the small cell size.

25. Type of mammogram, nominal

27. Nominal

29. Fail to reject the null, $p >$ alpha

31. Type two

33. No, this would be dependent samples and would require McNemar's test. Chi-square must have independent samples.

35. Nominal

37. Reject the null, $p <$ alpha

39. Because his screen is negative we know there is an 84% chance he does not have oropharyngeal cancer.

STUDENT *t*-TEST

HOW CAN I FIND A DIFFERENCE IN THE TWO SAMPLE MEANS IF MY DEPENDENT VARIABLE IS AT THE INTERVAL OR RATIO LEVEL?

OBJECTIVES

By the end of the chapter students will be able to:

- Identify the conditions under which the student *t*-test is an appropriate statistical technique.
- Compare and contrast dependent and independent samples.
- Identify independent and dependent samples in current nursing research.
- Write null and alternative hypotheses that demonstrate an understanding of the Student *t*-test.
- Calculate the degrees of freedom associated with a given data set.
- Interpret the SPSS output from a Student *t*-test, and determine whether it is

statistically significant; interpret this result in statistical terms and in plain English; and prepare a public health report using the information.

- Critique an article from current nursing research that utilizes the Student *t*-test; determine what type of sample was collected; identify whether the samples were independent or dependent; determine whether statistical significance is present; and debate whether clinical recommendations should be made.

KEY TERMS

Degrees of freedom for *t*-tests
Equals the sample size for both groups minus two.

Dependent samples
Paired or related groups or the same sample at a different time.

Independent samples
Do not have a relationship with one another.

Noninferiority trial
A trial used to show that a new treatment is no worse than an old procedure (may use a one-tailed test).

Sampling error
Error that occurs due to randomization and chance.

Student *t*-test
Used when you are looking for a difference in the mean value of an interval-level or a ratio-level variable.

THE STUDENT *T*-TEST

One of our favorite statistical tests is called the **Student *t*-test**, which was developed by William Gosset. Before you can apply the Student *t*-test to determine whether there is a difference between the means in the two sample groups, you need to determine three things:

- What is the level of measurement for the outcome variable?
- Are there two samples?
- Are the samples independent?

LEVEL OF MEASUREMENT

The Student *t*-test is appropriate only when you are looking for a difference in the mean value of an outcome variable that is at the interval or ratio level. In the next FTS we look at the difference in the amount of epinephrine in injectors, which is a ratio-level measurement (i.e., it shows a difference with equal ranked intervals and has a zero value), so it is appropriate.

The next question is what kind of samples do you have? First of all, are there two samples? To look for a difference in the mean value of the outcome variable, you must have at least two samples. In the injector example, you have a sample of injectors from Acme and a sample of injectors from EPI. So you have two samples, and you are looking for a difference in the mean amount of epinephrine found in each.

Now that you know you have two samples, you have to ask whether how you selected one sample affected the other. In the example, the two samples were randomly collected from two different kinds of injectors without any relationship to each other, so these are two **independent samples**. However, suppose you collected one sample of Acme injectors, measured their mean epinephrine levels preadministration, gave the injections, and then measured the residual epinephrine levels postadministration to see if there was a difference. (Obviously, if you are injecting the epinephrine there should be!) In that case, you would still have two samples, but they would be **dependent samples**, or related. Your second sample is a remeasurement of the same sample group at a different point in time.

You can also have dependent samples when you match sample characteristics. For example, if you are interested in comparing the average duration of hospital stay for individuals at two different hospitals, you might decide you want both samples to have been admitted for the same diagnosis. So you randomly sample 10 patients at the first hospital

FROM THE STATISTICIAN *Brendan Heavey*

Let's Talk *t*-Tests

Fueled by the success of scrubs sales by Carol's Nursing Scrubs, Carol has decided to expand her product offering to include injectable epinephrine pens. Carol has asked you to decide which type of pen she should retail. Two production companies are competing for the job: Acme Pens and EphedraPens International (EPI). They both produce injections that are advertised to hold 0.3 mg of epinephrine. The snag is that both companies have had some bad press recently over the amount of epinephrine in their products. Carol has asked you to check up on each company and decide whether one type of pen holds more epinephrine than the other.

In this scenario, you're interested in comparing the average amount of epinephrine in Acme's pens with the average amount of epinephrine in EPI's pens—two population parameters. The two companies are not going to give you access to their production facility to test out the whole population of pens, so you need to take a sample of each and make some inferences. Obviously, the samples from separate companies are independent of each other.

If it weren't for a man named William Gosset (1876–1937), answering questions like this would be much more difficult. After completing a degree at Oxford in 1899, Gosset decided to do what many other great Celtic men in history did and went to work for the Guinness brewery in Dublin, Ireland. While there, he was enlisted to work on projects to help decide how the quality of hops and barley affected the taste of a "pint o' the black stuff" (the proper way to refer to a glass of Guinness beer in Dublin). After Guinness sent him to study under a great statistician by the name of Karl Pearson, Gosset published a landmark paper that derived the *t*-distribution in 1908. Guinness considered his work top secret, and, as a result, he was forced to publish under the pen name "Student." This is why the *t*-distribution is sometimes referred to as "Student's *t*" or the Student *t*-test. This test is used when you are looking for a difference in the mean value of an interval- or a ratio-level variable.

Due to Gosset's work, we know we can perform an independent samples *t*-test on our epinephrine injection data to determine whether there is a statistical difference between the amounts of epinephrine in the two overall populations of injectors.

Note: All factual information regarding William Gosset was taken from Johnson and Kotz (1997).

and measure their length of stay. Then you go to the second hospital and randomly select 10 subjects with the same admission diagnosis as the first group. Because those selected for your second sample have to have had the same diagnosis as your first sample, they are not independent samples; they are correlated, or dependent. You can still determine whether the average length of stay differed depending on the hospital by comparing the mean from each group; however, to do this accurately, you have to use a *t*-test for dependent groups because that is the type of sample you have.

However, in the epinephrine injectors example, you know you have an outcome variable that is at the ratio level and two samples that are independent and randomly collected. The presence of these factors means that you can apply the Student *t*-test for independent groups. (Two other factors—normal distribution of the outcome variable and homogeneity of variance—are ideally also present, but they are not absolutely essential, even though they do impact statistical interpretation. You can explore these factors more fully in the upcoming From the Statistician section.)

So, before applying an independent Student *t*-test, simply answer the following questions:

- Is my outcome variable at the interval or ratio level?
- Do I have two samples?
- Are my samples random and independent from one another?

If your answers to these three questions are yes, you may proceed with a Student *t*-test for independent groups.

THE NULL AND ALTERNATIVE HYPOTHESES

In the example, the null hypothesis is that there is no difference between the mean amounts of epinephrine in the two types of epinephrine injectors. Our alternative hypothesis, therefore, is that there is a difference between the mean amounts of epinephrine in the two types of pens. We collect our first sample of pens from Acme and find that the average amount of epinephrine in each injector is 0.31 mg. We then collect our second sample of pens from EPI and find the average amount is 0.30 mg. There is a difference in the sample means, but is it statistically significant or is it just due to **sampling error** (error that occurs due to randomization and chance)? Because this appears to be a relatively small difference between the means, it is unlikely to be significant, but remember that it could be if the sample size is large.

STATISTICAL SIGNIFICANCE

To determine whether the difference is statistically significant, you have to decide on a number of things:

- *The level of risk you are going to take that you will incorrectly reject the null hypothesis (alpha):* For this example, you decide to take a 5% chance that you will make a type one error, so you select an alpha of 0.05.
- *The power (the chance of finding a difference if it actually exists):* You decide that 0.80, or 80%, is adequate.
- *Whether you are conducting a one-tailed or two-tailed test:* These terms simply indicate whether you are looking for

a difference in either direction (two-tailed) or you have hypothesized that the difference is in a specific direction, such as the mean in the second sample is greater than or less than the mean in the first (one-tailed). Because this example is looking for a difference in any direction between the epinephrine levels in the two groups, you are going to do a two-tailed Student *t*-test.

FROM THE STATISTICIAN *Brendan Heavey*

Using a One-Tailed Test

Using a one-sided, or one-tailed, hypothesis test is a controversial procedure that should be avoided in most instances. A researcher who is interested in a *directional* null hypothesis would use a one-tailed test. The assumption is that, based on prior information or previous testing, there is no chance of a change in one of the two possible directions for a particular variable. Therefore, alpha (*a*), which is usually split between two tails, has its probability shifted to one tail (or one side), as we see in **Figure 9-1**.

One-tailed tests are sometimes acceptable. Their most common use is in **noninferiority trials**, whose point is to show that a new treatment is no worse than an old procedure. For example, a new noninvasive procedure is found that might be a replacement for an older invasive procedure. We don't want to show that the new procedure is better than the old one, only that it is no worse. In this case, using a one-tailed test makes sense because the probability in the *upper* or right side of the tail would indicate that our new noninvasive procedure performed better than our old procedure. Because there is virtually no likelihood of this occurring, we shift the probability to the *lower* or left side of the tail. In this case, we are testing the following null and alternative hypotheses:

H_0: There is no difference between the two therapies.
H_1: The change in response from one therapy is *less than* the change in response from another.

If we were using a two-tailed test, the alternative hypothesis would look like this:

H_1: The change in response from one therapy is different from the change in response from another.

Can you see the difference between these two alternative hypotheses?

Some researchers overuse one-tailed tests. Why is this practice a problem? Can you figure out why we cannot use one-tailed tests all the time? Is it easier or more difficult to attain statistical significance with a one-tailed test? Let's look at a scenario in which a one-sided test is inappropriate.

Let's say you are working for a pharmaceutical company that has discovered a new drug to treat the flu. The drug is suspected to reduce fever, so your company has you test this hypothesis with the following procedure:

- Enroll 200 subjects who have the flu.
- Administer the test drug to 100 subjects and a placebo sugar pill to the other 100.
- Wait 4 hours and then take everyone's temperature.

(continues)

FROM THE STATISTICIAN *Brendan Heavey*

In this case, let's say we use a two-sample Student *t*-test to test the difference between average temperatures in these two groups 4 hours after they take the test or placebo pill. You end up with data as shown in **Figure 9-2**.

The corresponding *p*-value is not significant when we use a two-tailed test, but it is if we use a one-tailed test.

If you are working for the drug company that is pressing to get this new drug to market, you might use a one-sided test based on the argument that there is no chance the new drug will increase fever. Switching to a one-sided test would be a violation of a number of issues, however: You did not decide which test you were going to use beforehand, and you have no prior research to suggest that the pill could not elevate a fever. Needless to say, using a one-tailed test in this situation is not advisable. In fact, one-tailed testing is so frowned upon that some scientific journals require only two-sided *p*-values to be reported. This policy is in place to prevent researchers from cheating and attaining statistical significance in their work too easily.

For examples of appropriate one-sided tests in the literature, see:

- *The Diamond trial:* A noninvasive ultrasound procedure was tested against amniocentesis, an older and more invasive procedure, to test for severe fetal anemia (Oepkes, 2006).
- *Neuroblastoma screening:* Researchers investigated whether neuroblastoma screening in infancy improved the survival of children diagnosed with this disease (Schilling, 2002).
- *Effect of lidocaine during breast biopsy:* Researchers determined that applying topical lidocaine decreased the pain women experienced during breast biopsy (Olbrys, 2001).

DEGREES OF FREEDOM FOR STUDENT *T*-TESTS

This test involves one other concept: **degrees of freedom**, which is equal to the sample size for both groups minus two. This is the same as taking the degrees of freedom for each group (sample size for the group minus one) and adding them together. Now you might feel as though you have no freedom, but in your study you do; let's see how much. When you collect a sample of 10 injectors and measure their epinephrine levels, you have 10 values that are "free" to vary depending on which injectors you select and how much epinephrine is in

each. However, once you calculate the mean level of epinephrine, only nine of the values are actually free to be "unknown" at any one time. Once you know the amount of epinephrine in each of the nine injector pens and you know the mean, you can figure out how much epinephrine is in the last injector. The value for the last injector pen is no longer free to vary; so when you calculate the mean, you lose a degree of freedom.

If degrees of freedom still has you totally baffled, just remember this: Take your total sample size (both groups) minus two (one from each group), and you know the degrees

| FIGURE 9-1 | **Location of Alpha (a) With a Two-Sided versus One-Sided Test.** |

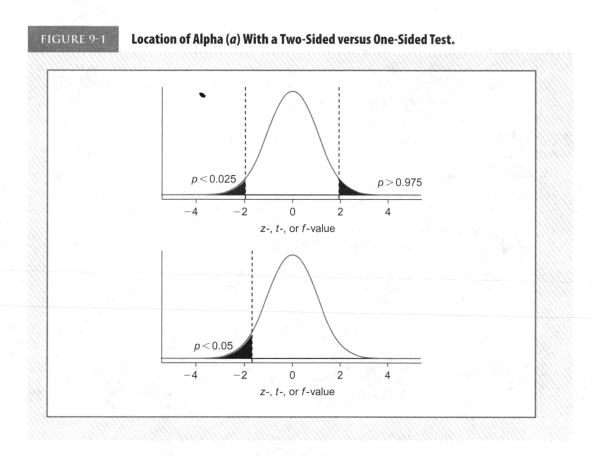

| FIGURE 9-2 | **Clinical Trial for a New Flu Medication.** |

	Average Temperature After
Drug	101.2
Placebo	102.1

of freedom for the test which is all you need to then find the corresponding p-value on a t-distribution table (see **Figure 9-3**).

(You can still perform a Student t-test without really understanding this concept. Just don't tell the statisticians I said so!)

So when are we getting to the really exciting Student *t*-test? The reality of nursing work today is that you won't be making the calculation. However, for those of you who really want to see the equation, you can check it out in the next From the Statistician: Methods. All the rest of you need only to be able to look at a computer printout or a research article and understand what it means.

| FIGURE 9-3 | **Formula for Calculating Degrees of Freedom for Student *t*-Tests.** |

$$\text{Degrees of freedom} = (n_1 + n_2) - 2$$

where
n_1 = total number of subjects in sample one
n_2 = total number of subjects in sample two

FROM THE STATISTICIAN *Brendan Heavey*

Methods: Student's *t*-Test

Student's *t*-test is so named because it makes use of what is called the *t*-statistical distribution. The test is probably the most often used statistical test, for better or worse. I say "for better or worse" because it is not always the correct test to run; it is just usually the most straightforward.

The purpose of a two-sample *t*-test is to determine whether the means of two groups differ significantly.

The *t*-test has a few versions, so you have to ask a few questions before performing one:

1. *How many tails (one or two) of the statistical distribution do you want to test?* For an in-depth discussion of this topic, see the For the Statistician: Using a One-Tailed Test earlier in the chapter.
2. *Is your data paired?* In some instances, data is set up so that the two groups under consideration have members that are paired instead of being independent. An example of paired data occurs in a so-called crossover clinical trial, in which subjects are given both a placebo and a drug (as shown in **Figure 9-4**). Setting up a trial in this manner is suitable for a paired analysis because each subject has two measures taken: one with the placebo and one with the drug. Because these measures are not measured on two different subjects, the *t*-test that compares their outcomes must be adjusted to account for their nonindependence, and a repeated measures test for the difference in dependent samples should be used.

(continues)

FROM THE STATISTICIAN *Brendan Heavey*

3. *Can you assume equal variances in the two different groups?* One of the assumptions of the two-sample *t*-test is that the two groups have the same variance. Slight departures from this assumption are okay, but if they are too extreme, a different formula should be used. (That alternative is beyond the scope of this text.) Statisticians describe this property as homogeneity of variance or equal variances. (You can try out that vocabulary at your next racquetball match!)

Here is an example of an independent-sample *t*-test to determine if there is a difference in the mean age between two mutually exclusive groups. Data was collected on trauma cases ages 25 and younger during one 72-hour period at an upstate New York tertiary care facility. We were interested in comparing the mean ages between groups who did have a positive drug screen and those who did not. The data set used is shown in **Figure 9-5**. We ran a basic analysis in SPSS, whose output is shown in **Figures 9-6** through **9-10**.

Is the homogeneity of variance assumption appropriate to use in this case? Let's look at the standard deviations of the two groups. We see that the drug-screen-negative group has a standard deviation of 8.54593, whereas the drug-screen-positive group has a standard deviation of 3.28634 (**Figure 9-9**). Tests are available that can be used to decide whether the equivariance assumption holds. The SPSS we chose used Levene's test for equality of variances. Note the large discrepancy in the standard deviations compared to their overall magnitude; we can agree that they are pretty far off from each other. Levene's test for equality of variances tests the null hypothesis that the variances in the two groups are not different. In this example, the Levene's test for equality of variances has a significant *p*-value, so you reject the null hypothesis that the variances are equal and use the second line of the *t*-test analysis (for when equal variances are not assumed). That line shows a *t*-value of -1.294, which converts to a two-tailed *p*-value of 0.212. Because the study had an alpha of 0.05, you know that this *p*-value is not adequate to reject H_0. Therefore, you fail to reject H_0: There is not enough evidence to suggest there is a difference in the mean ages of patients in the two groups of a positive and a negative drug screen.

Let's look at a brief computation that explains what makes up the *t*-value. If the standard deviations for the two groups were similar and we therefore assumed equal variances, you would calculate the appropriate *t*-value (T) by means of the following formula:

$$T = \frac{\bar{X}_1 - \bar{X}_2}{SE}$$

The difference between the sample means ($\bar{X}_1 - \bar{X}_2$) was -3.42857, and the standard error (SE) of the difference, assuming equal variances, was 3.64319; so, the calculation looks like this:

$$\frac{-3.42857}{3.64319} = -0.941$$

Notice that -0.941 is the *t*-value associated with the test on the statistical computing output table (**Figure 9-10**). If you did not assume equal variances, the denominator would be the standard error of the difference of 2.64, and the resulting *t*-value would be -1.294 (see **Figure 9-10**).

FROM THE STATISTICIAN *Brendan Heavey*

FIGURE 9-4   **Crossover Study Design.**

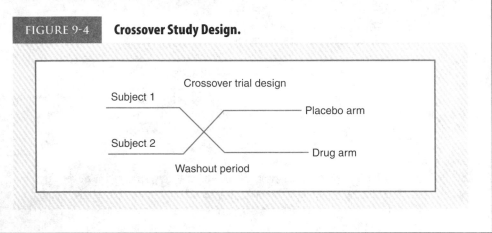

FIGURE 9-5   **Age and Drug Screen Status for Patients Under Age 25 in a Trauma Center.**

Age	Drug Screen	Age	Drug Screen
2	0	20	0
3	0	20	1
5	0	20	1
7	0	21	1
8	0	22	0
15	1	22	0
15	1	23	1
18	0	23	0
19	0	25	0
19	0	25	0

Drug screen: 0 = negative, 1 = positive

| FIGURE 9-6 | **Frequency Table for Age.** |

Age

	Frequency	Percentage	Valid Percentage	Cumulative Percentage
Valid 2	1	5.0	5.0	5.0
3	1	5.0	5.0	10.0
5	1	5.0	5.0	15.0
7	1	5.0	5.0	20.0
8	1	5.0	5.0	25.0
15	2	10.0	10.0	35.0
18	1	5.0	5.0	40.0
19	2	10.0	10.0	50.0
20	3	15.0	15.0	65.0
21	1	5.0	5.0	70.0
22	2	10.0	10.0	80.0
23	2	10.0	10.0	90.0
25	2	10.0	10.0	100.0
Total	20	100.0	100.0	

| FIGURE 9-7 | **Descriptive Statistics for Age Variable.** |

N	Valid	20.0000
	Missing	0.0000
Mean		16.6000
Median		19.5000
Mode		20.0000

(continues)

FIGURE 9-7   **Descriptive Statistics for Age Variable.**

Standard deviation		7.4438
Variance		55.4105
Skewness		−0.9158
Standard error of skewness		0.5121
Percentiles	25	9.7500
	50	19.5000
	75	22.0000

FIGURE 9-8   **Bar Chart for Age Variable.**

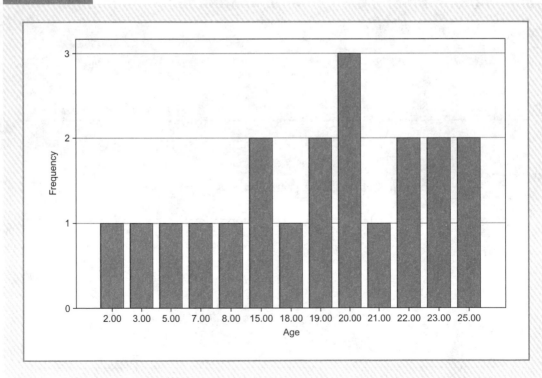

FIGURE 9-9	**Means by Drug Screen Status.**

Group Statistics

Drug Screen		*N*	Mean	Standard Deviation	Standard Error Mean
Age	Negative	14	15.5714	8.54593	2.28400
	Positive	6	19.0000	3.28634	1.34164

FIGURE 9-10	***t*-Test for Equality of Mean Age Between Those With a Negative and Those With a Positive Drug Screen.**

Independent Samples Test

		Levene's Test for Equality of Variances		*t*-Test for Equality of Means							
										95% Confidence Interval of the Difference	
		F	Significance	*t*	*df*	Significance (two-tailed)	Mean Difference	Standard Error Difference	Lower	Upper
Age	Equal variances assumed	11.098	0.004	−0.941	18	0.359	−3.42857	3.64319	−11.08264	4.22550
	Equal variances not assumed			−1.294	17.960	0.212	−3.42857	2.64889	−8.99459	2.13745

SUMMARY

You have just completed this chapter. Very impressive! Now let's review the main points.

First and foremost, remember that the null hypothesis is that there is no difference between the group means. The Student *t*-test is used to determine whether there is a difference in an interval- or a ratio-level outcome or dependent variable in two sample groups. If the sample groups are independent, the sample groups do not have any relationship. If the samples are dependent, the groups are matched on an attribute or may be the same group measured at a different time; in either case they are related to each other. The sampling error occurs due to randomization or chance, and the degrees of freedom equal the total sample size minus two.

CHAPTER 9 REVIEW QUESTIONS

Questions 1–11: You are asked to design a study determining whether there is a difference in the average fasting blood glucose for individuals with diabetes randomized either to a strictly dietary intervention or to a diet and exercise intervention.

1. Are you looking for a relationship/association or a difference?

2. What is your dependent variabe?

3. Is it qualitative or quantitative? Is it continuous or categorical? What level of measurement is it?

4. How many samples do you have? Is this a probability or nonprobability sampling method?

5. Are these independent or dependent groups?

6. Would you prefer to use a chi-square test or a Student *t*-test with this study?

7. Write appropriate null and alternative hypotheses.
   Null:

   Alternative:

8. Your study includes an alpha of 0.05 and a power of 0.80. You conduct a Student *t*-test, which has a *p*-value of 0.07. What is your conclusion?

9. What type of error might you be making?

10. A trial is repeated with a larger sample and the Student *t*-test has a *p*-value of 0.04. What is your conclusion now?

_____

_____

11. What type of error might you be making now?

_____

Questions 12–24: Chung and Hwang (2008) examined the difference between an experimental and a control group of patients with leukemia. The experimental group received two follow-up phone calls after discharge, and the control group received routine care. Their Table 2 is reproduced as **Figure 9-11**.

12. What was the independent variable?

_____

13. What were the dependent variables?

_____

_____

14. What was the mean score for the quality of life for each group?

_____

_____

15. Which group had a higher quality of life 4 weeks after discharge? Was this statistically significant?

_____

_____

FIGURE 9-11   **Test of Two-Group Differences 4 Weeks After Discharge.**

Variable	Experimental Group (N = 35)		Control Group (N = 35)		
	X	*SD*	*X*	*SD*	*t*
Self-care	2.67	0.36	1.78	0.38	10.347*
Symptom distress	0.34	0.21	0.82	0.51	−5.158*
Quality of life	70.46	18.76	44.15	16.01	6.074*

*$p < 0.001$

Source: Oncology nursing forum by ONCOLOGY NURSING SOCIETY. Reproduced with permission of ONCOLOGY NURSING SOCIETY in the format Republish in a book via Copyright Clearance Center.

16. What was the mean score for self-care for each group?

_____

_____

17. Which group had the ability to provide more of its own self-care? Was this a statistically significant difference?

_____

_____

18. Which group had a higher level of symptom distress? Was this statistically significant?

_____

_____

19. Interpret these findings in plain English, and give a plausible explanation for them.

_____

_____

_____

20. Look at **Figure 9-12** from the same study. Interpret the statistically significant results in plain English.

_____

_____

_____

21. Did the experimental group have higher levels of any symptom of distress?

_____

22. A convenience sample was used. Is this a probability or nonprobability sampling method?

_____

23. How might this affect the results?

_____

24. How could you improve on this study's sampling method?

_____

Questions 25–31: You are conducting a small study at your hospital looking at infants born in the first 24 hours after the conclusion of a hurricane. You classify prematurity status as full term (0) if the infants are born after 37 weeks of gestation and premature (1) if they are born before 37 weeks of gestation. You measure birth weight in grams at the time of delivery. You conduct a *t*-test to see whether the mean birth weights differ between the premature and full-term infants. See **Figures 9-13** and **9-14**.

25. What is your sample size?

_____

26. What is the mean birth weight for full-term infants?

_____

FIGURE 9-12	**Test of Two-Group Differences of Symptom Distress.**

Variable	Experimental Group (N=35)		Control Group (N=35)		t
	X	SD	X	SD	
Appetite change	1.00	1.59	1.66	1.24	−1.931
Fatigue	1.00	0.59	2.11	1.13	−5.158***
Appearance change	1.14	1.03	1.54	1.15	−1.533
Nausea	0.43	0.61	0.46	0.74	0.464
Irritability	0.29	0.46	0.86	0.73	−3.909***
Change in sexual interest	0.71	0.83	1.23	1.17	−2.131
Insomnia (sleeplessness)	0.17	0.38	1.09	1.20	−4.303***
Dry mouth	0.34	0.48	1.23	1.06	−4.502***
Pain	0.37	0.65	0.97	1.22	−2.564
Dizziness	0.43	0.65	0.51	0.78	−0.498
Lack of concentration	0.23	0.43	0.94	0.87	−4.325***
Numbness	0.26	0.44	0.83	0.79	−3.748***
Diarrhea	—	—	0.29	0.52	−3.260**
Chest discomfort	0.09	0.37	0.43	0.70	−2.562*
Oral or esophageal ulcer	0.26	0.44	0.49	0.89	−1.364
Stomach discomfort	0.09	0.28	0.23	0.49	−1.492
Dyspnea	0.11	0.40	1.02	3.57	−1.506
Bleeding	0.11	0.40	0.49	0.92	−2.188*
Cough	0.17	0.38	0.60	0.81	−2.826*
Trembling	0.09	0.37	0.43	0.74	−2.449*
Fever	0.06	0.24	0.40	0.74	−2.626*
Dysuria	0.09	0.37	0.14	0.69	−0.430

*$p < 0.05$; **$p < 0.01$; ***$p < 0.001$

FIGURE 9-13 **Mean Birth Weight for Full-Term and Premature Infants.**

Group Statistics

Preterm Status		I	Mean	Standard Deviation	Standard Error Mean
Birth weight	0	6	3453.3333	435.41551	177.75764
	1	4	1225.0000	357.07142	178.53571

FIGURE 9-14 ***t*-Test for Equality of Mean Birth Weight in Full-Term and Premature Infants.**

Independent Samples Test

		Levene's Test for Equality of Variances		*t*-Test for Equality of Means						95% Confidence Interval of the Difference	
		F	Significance	*t*	df	Significance (two-tailed)	Mean Difference	Standard Error Difference		Lower	Upper
Birth weight	Equal variances assumed	0.767	0.407	8.465	8	0.000	2228.33333	253.23640		1621.30910	2835.35756
	Equal variances not assumed			7.484		0.000	2228.33333	251.93804		1640.30927	2816.35740

27. What is the mean birth weight for preterm infants?

_____

28. Which group has a larger standard deviation?

_____

29. Because the Levene's test for equality of variances is not significant, the standard practice is to assume equal variances. What is the appropriate *t*-value?

_____

30. Is the *t*-value significant?

_____

31. What do you conclude?

_____

FROM THE STATISTICIAN REVIEW QUESTION

32. The appropriate *t*-value when not assuming equal variances has been removed from the table in Figure 9-14. Calculate what it would be.

Questions 33–40: A researcher in a Veterans Affairs hospital wants to determine whether patients who had metal-on-metal hardware vs. ceramic-on-metal hardware used for their hip replacements have different levels of chromium ions (measured in mcg/mL or parts per billion [ppb] from 0 and up) in their blood 2 years later. A sample of all patients who had full hip replacements with these two types of hardware at the hospital in the last 2 years is collected for a total of 145 subjects in the study. The researcher sets her alpha at 0.05 and her power at 0.80.

_____

33. What is the dependent variable in the study?

_____

34. If serum chromium levels are measured in mcg/mL what level of measurement is this variable?

_____

_____

35. Would you recommend using a chi-square or an independent *t*-test to answer this question? Why?

_____

36. What type of sample is this? Is it a probability or nonprobability sample?

_____

_____

37. The average serum chromium in the metal-on-metal group is 0.78 ppb and the average serum chromium in the ceramic-on-metal hardware group is 0.45. The *t*-test results have a *p*-value of 0.043. What conclusion should the researcher draw about the null hypothesis? Why?

_____

38. In this study the researcher also compares these two groups to see if the type of hardware utilized for the hip replacement results in differing average Harris Hip functionality scores 6 months postop (scored from 0–100). What is the independent variable and what level of measurement is this variable?

_____

_____

39. The results in this portion of the analysis have a *p*-value of 0.27. What should the researcher conclude about the null hypothesis for this portion of the study?

_____

_____

40. The researcher later discovers that the effect size for the difference in the Harris Hip functionality is much smaller than she had anticipated. She is now concerned she may have made what type of error in this portion of the study?

_____

_____

ANSWERS TO CHAPTER 9 REVIEW QUESTIONS

1. Difference

3. Quantitative, continuous, interval/ratio

5. Independent

7. Answers may vary, for example: H_0: There is no difference in fasting blood glucose in the diet–only group versus the diet and exercise group. H_1: There is a difference in the fasting blood glucose for the two groups.

9. Type two

11. Type one

13. Self-care, symptom distress, quality of life

15. Experimental, yes

17. Experimental, yes

19. Telephone support worked, or the experimental group was just healthier. (They had lower signs and symptoms of distress, and there was nonrandom assignment and no pretest, so we don't know whether this group was just healthier to start with.)

21. No

23. The groups may have been significantly different before the intervention.

25. 10

27. 1225 g

29. 8.465

31. Reject the null. There is a significant difference in the mean age of premature infants and full-term infants in this sample.

33. Serum chromium mcg/mL or ppb

35. *t*-Test because there are two independent samples and an outcome or dependent variable at the ratio level

37. Reject the null, $p <$ alpha, the metal-on-metal group has a significantly higher average serum chromium level.

39. Fail to reject the null, $p >$ alpha.

ANALYSIS OF VARIANCE (ANOVA)

HOW DO I COMPARE THE DEPENDENT VARIABLE MEANS FROM MORE THAN TWO SAMPLES?

OBJECTIVES

By the end of the chapter students will be able to:

- Describe the conditions in which ANOVA would be an appropriate test.
- Write null and alternative hypotheses that demonstrate understanding of the guiding principles of ANOVA.
- Determine whether ANOVA test results are significant.
- Describe ANOVA study results in plain English.
- Compare ANOVA and repeat-measures ANOVA.

- Relate situations in which repeat-measures ANOVA would be useful and explain why.
- Express some limitations or concerns associated with repeat-measures ANOVA.
- Critique a current nursing research article that uses ANOVA and interpret the results statistically and in plain English; and prepare a public health report using this information.

KEY TERMS

ANOVA (analysis of variance)
The test used when comparing the means from a single dependent variable among two or more groups or samples.

Carry-over effects
Occur when previous treatments continue to have an effect through the next treatment, affecting the measurement of the dependent variable.

Compound symmetry
Measurements are correlated and of equal variances.

Homogeneity of variance
Equal variances among the groups being compared.

Position or latency effects
Occur when a subject is being exposed to more than one treatment over time and the order of the treatment received impacts the outcome.

Power
Probability of detecting a difference that really exists.

Repeat-measures ANOVA
Examines a change over time in the same sample population.

COMPARING MORE THAN TWO SAMPLES

When performing a study, there is a test to find a difference between two groups when you have an outcome variable that is a nominal or an ordinal level of measurement (chi-square test), and another if you have an outcome variable that is an interval or a ratio level of measurement (*t*-test). But both of these methods assume you are examining the differences between only two independent samples. What if you have more than two samples or groups? You could do multiple *t*-tests, but you could compare only two groups at a time, and each comparison would have a risk of a type one error equal to alpha (e.g., 0.05). Even doing three *t*-tests to compare three groups (1 + 2, 2 + 3, 1 + 3) increases the risk of a type one error to 0.05 + 0.05 + 0.05, or 0.15, which is substantial.

For this reason, statisticians prefer to use a different test called **analysis of variance (ANOVA)** when comparing more than two groups or sample means.

THE NULL AND ALTERNATIVE HYPOTHESES

Suppose you are working on a study to examine the average systolic blood pressure of men from different racial groups. Your sample includes subjects who are Caucasian (group 1), African American (group 2), and Latino (group 3). Your null hypothesis is that all the men will have a similar mean systolic blood pressure regardless of racial background.

$$H_0: M_1 = M_2 = M_3$$

The alternative hypothesis is:

H_1: The three means are not equal.

Note: They don't all have to be unequal. Even if two are significantly unequal, you would reject the null hypothesis.

The analysis of variance test determines whether the differences seen in the sample means are significantly larger than one would expect by mere chance. An equation then produces an *F*-ratio that relates the differences between the groups (the numerator) to the difference within the groups (the denominator). (For those of you who are interested, check out the From the Statistician: Methods box at the end of the chapter. You can study the equation to your heart's content.)

When the null hypothesis is correct and there is not a difference in the means of the groups being studied, the *F*-ratio is close to 1. In that case, the differences between the groups are very similar to the differences within the groups (due to normal individual differences), and the *F*-ratio is not significant.

DEGREES OF FREEDOM

As usual, there is also a measure of degrees of freedom. The difference is that the numerator of the *F*-ratio has one number for degrees of freedom (number of groups minus one) and the denominator of the *F*-ratio has another (the number of subjects minus the number of groups). When you add the two, the sum becomes the degrees of freedom associated with the *F*-ratio.

STATISTICAL SIGNIFICANCE

The *F*-ratio is like any other statistical measure in that it has a *p*-value that determines its significance. You can look up the *p*-value on a table for the *F*-distribution, or you can just program your statistical computing package to tell you what it is. If the *p*-value is less than the alpha you select (e.g., 0.05), then you have the statistical strength to reject the null hypothesis and report that there is a difference among the average blood pressures of the three samples or groups. If, on the other hand, you have an alpha of 0.05 and your *F*-ratio has a *p*-value of 0.09, you must fail to reject the null and conclude that you do not have the statistical power to show a difference or that there really isn't one.

In your study of systolic blood pressure in men from different racial groups, let's say you find that the average for group 1 is 142, group 2's is 145, and group 3's is 128. Your *F*-ratio has a *p*-value of 0.02, and your alpha is 0.05. You therefore reject the null hypothesis and conclude that there are differences among the mean systolic blood pressures of these three racial groups. When you report these results, you need to include what the means are for each group and that there is a statistical difference.

You cannot conclude from this test alone where the statistically significant difference may lie. Perhaps group 2 was significantly greater than group 3 but not significantly greater than group 1. Perhaps there was a significant difference among all three groups. You would need to do further testing to draw that conclusion. This test merely lets you conclude that there is a difference among the average blood pressures of men from different racial groups.

If you really want to impress someone at your next holiday party show them an analysis of variance test with only two groups (remember you could just do a *t*-test for that!) and then determine the *F*-ratio. If you take the square root, you have the *t*-value, which you could have determined by just doing a *t*-test on the two groups. It is statistically acceptable, but not necessary, to compute an *F*-ratio from an ANOVA test when there are only two groups and you will reach the same conclusion as you would using the *t*-test. All of this might not be great dinner conversation, but it might come in handy the next time you are trying to discourage a boring hanger-on.

FROM THE STATISTICIAN *Brendan Heavey*

Relationship Between Distributions

What is the relationship among chi-square analyses, *t*-tests, and *F*-tests? The following three facts might surprise you:

1. If an ANOVA analysis is performed on just two groups of subjects, the test gives the same results as a *t*-test.
2. The *t*-distribution, which is the underlying probability distribution of the *t*-test, looks almost identical to the normal distribution. In fact, the only difference is that it is a little flatter, with more probability assigned to the tails of the distribution.
3. An easy way to produce a chi-squared distribution is by summing the squares of a series of standard normal variables.

There are standard ways of converting among these distributions. The math is a bit higher level than we want to discuss here, but it is certainly doable. The process is called *transformation*. Some transformations are quite simple, like the square root transformation performed by taking the square root of every data point in a study variable. Other transformations are quite difficult and can involve formulas longer than a page.

Often, students feel discouraged in introductory statistics classes because they have a difficult time with the properties of distributions and the relationships between them. If you choose to go on to another statistics course (or if you are forced to take another one because of degree requirements), keep in mind the fact that they are all related. Perhaps this insight will give you a bit more motivation to understand their intricacies.

You can choose from an unlimited number of probability distributions. They all must have a total sum of probability, or area under the curve, equal to 1. Whenever you have to deal with a new one, just remember the five-step process for statistical testing, and you should be all right. In fact, you can do a surprising amount of decent statistical analysis by learning how to use a basic statistical software package like SPSS. You can thank the great statistical minds that came before us, like Pearson, R.A. Fisher, and Samuel Gosset, for figuring out all the equations for you!

APPROPRIATE USE OF ANOVA

Several assumptions should be met before you use ANOVA.

-   First, the samples must be independent (ideally random), and the measure must be at the interval or ratio level.

-   The sample should have a normal distribution—but remember the central limit theorem. Because we are comparing means, we can comfortably assume normality. The distribution of the original population doesn't matter; the means will be normally distributed.

- The last assumption is **homogeneity of variance**, which also is not terribly concerning at this level because ANOVA still works pretty well even if this assumption is not met.

So the big takeaway message about assumptions and ANOVA is that you need independent samples with an outcome or a dependent variable at the interval or ratio level. You don't have to be too concerned about the other assumptions. You should know about them, however, because you will see your statistics computing program assess them (Norman & Streiner, 2008).

REPEAT-MEASURES ANOVA

ANOVA has another really exciting application. (I can see you jumping out of your seats with excitement now! But please remain calm). It is called **repeat-measures ANOVA**, and it is useful for dependent samples. You will see this application used frequently in nursing literature that examines a change over time in the same sample population. For example, suppose you want to compare the mean body mass index (BMI) of a group of children who participated in a 12-week after-school basketball program and a comparison group who did not. BMI becomes your dependent variable, and you are going to measure it, in each of the subjects and the controls, before the subjects begin the program, halfway through the program, and upon completion of the program. You can also design a study appropriate for repeat-measures ANOVA by taking the same group of subjects and measuring their weights before any intervention, then giving them three different weight control interventions, one at a time with 2 weeks per intervention. You then measure their weights before and after each intervention. By repeating the measures on the same group of subjects, you create a level of control over differences among the participants and make it easier to isolate the differences resulting from your intervention. You thus increase the likelihood that you will find statistically significant results when they exist. In effect, you increase the (can you hear the drum roll here?) **power** of the study (or the ability to detect a difference that really exists). You saw that coming, right?

ISSUES OF CONCERN WITH REPEAT-MEASURES ANOVA

Repeat-measures ANOVA can be very helpful in decreasing not only the individual variation error, but also the required sample size needed to find a significant result. This is particularly helpful when it is difficult to recruit subjects or when funding is difficult to obtain.

However, all researchers using this method need to be aware of a couple of concerns:

- **Position or latency effects** occur when a subject is being exposed to more than one treatment over time and the order of the treatment received impacts the outcome. For example, let's say you have a cancer study that includes treatment with surgery and chemotherapy. If surgically removing the cancerous tumor improves the ability of the chemotherapy to eliminate any remaining cancer cells, subjects who start with the surgery, followed by the chemotherapy, may experience a greater effect than those who start with the chemotherapy followed by the surgery. You can address this concern by randomly assigning the order of the interventions.

- **Carry-over effects** occur when previous treatments continue to have an effect through the next treatment. In this case, the measurement of the outcome or dependent variable after a particular treatment does not just reflect the impact of that treatment but rather includes the additional effect from the previous treatment as well. For example, if subjects in a weight study take a diet pill with a long half-life, they may need a "wash-out" period before beginning the next intervention to avoid having the effect of two interventions at the same time (Plichta & Garzon, 2009).

APPROPRIATE USE OF REPEAT-MEASURES ANOVA

Like all other statistical techniques, appropriate use of repeat-measures ANOVA involves meeting some basic assumptions. Most of the assumptions are the same as those for ANOVA, but there is one more—**compound symmetry**. Compound symmetry means that the measurements are correlated and of equal variances. So, if you are measuring BMI three times, the three results should be correlated with one another and approximately the same. Homogeneity of variance should also still be present and is the term used to indicate that those correlated BMI measurements need to have approximately equal variances.

The good news is that, once again, your statistical computing package will check all of this for you. If you look at your SPSS output, you will see an area for Mauchly's sphericity test. If this test is not significant, you can tell the assumption of compound symmetry is met and can proceed with your analysis confidently (Munro, 2005). What on earth did we do before SPSS? Okay, I have to admit, I remember—and it wasn't pretty.

FROM THE STATISTICIAN *Brendan Heavey*

Methods: Calculating an *F*-Statistic

An analysis of variance is a lot like a *t*-test extended to multiple groups of data. It is a little more difficult to understand conceptually, but in my opinion well worth the effort to learn! In fact, if you don't use ANOVA, you sometimes have to do a whole series of *t*-tests, and that can quickly increase the error associated with your analysis.

Let's say we have two variables; one is continuous and one is categorical. The categorical variable has three levels, and we are interested in looking at the mean value of the continuous variable in each of these categories. (See **Figure 10-1**.) Each of the three cells in the table has its own mean, which is identified using the Greek letter μ (mu). (Don't ask me why we use ancient Greek; we follow the mathematicians' lead on this.) Attached to each μ character is a subscript that indicates the number of the group from which the mean is determined. The overall mean (or grand mean) is denoted by a period (μ). In ANOVA, we are always interested in a null hypothesis that makes all of the individual cell means equal to one another.

To perform a test of this hypothesis, we compute an *F*-statistic (named after R.A. Fisher, who developed ANOVA). The *F*-statistic is simply a ratio of variances. (Remember, variance is just a measure of how a set of values differs from a

(continues)

FROM THE STATISTICIAN *Brendan Heavey*

FIGURE 10-1   **Beginning of General ANOVA Table.**

	Level 1	Level 2	Level 3	Grand Mean
Variable	μ_1	μ_2	μ_3	μ

single value.) The first variance component in an *F*-statistic is derived from the variance of the cell means around the grand mean. (This is the variance between the groups.) The second variance component in an *F*-statistic is derived from how each individual data point differs from its respective cell mean. (This is the variance within the group itself.)

Let's look at an example. We collected data on trauma cases ages 25 and younger during one 72-hour period at an upstate New York tertiary care facility. We then compared the mean age between groups who had a positive drug screen and those who did not. Now we are interested in seeing whether the mean age of a patient differs among the classes of injury the patients had treated. The data is presented in **Figure 10-2**.

The first step is to get our data to look like the generalized table (**Figure 10-3**). **Figure 10-4** shows how our data looks in the general ANOVA table.

Now we solve for the unknown parameters:

$$\mu_1 = \frac{5+25}{2} = 15$$

$$\mu_2 = \frac{7+19+20+23+23}{5} = 18.4$$

$$\mu_3 = \frac{2+2+8+15+15+18+19+20+20+21+22+22+25}{13} = 16.08$$

$$\mu = \frac{5+25+7+19+20+23+23+2+2+8+15+15+18+19+20+20+21+22+22+25}{20} = 16.6$$

In this hypothesis, our null hypothesis is:

H_0: The three *cell means,* $\mu_1 = 15, \mu_2 = 18.4, \mu_3 = 16.08$, are equal.

The alternative hypothesis is:
  H_1: They are not *all* equal.

(continues)

FROM THE STATISTICIAN *Brendan Heavey*

FIGURE 10-2   **Age and Injury Level for Patients Seen in a 72-hour Period at a Trauma Center.**

Age	Injury	Age	Injury
2	2	20	1
3	2	20	2
5	0	20	2
7	1	20	2
8	2	22	2
15	2	22	2
15	2	23	1
18	2	23	1
19	1	25	0
19	2	25	2

FIGURE 10-3   **Setting up a General ANOVA Table for Age and Injury Example.**

	Factor Level 1	Factor Level 2	Factor Level 3	Grand Mean
Variable	μ_1	μ_2	μ_3	μ

The results of the ANOVA are shown in **Figure 10-5**. The p-value for this test is 0.823, derived from the F-statistic value of 0.198. Assuming an alpha of 0.05, this p-value indicates that there is not enough evidence to reject the null hypothesis.

(continues)

FROM THE STATISTICIAN *Brendan Heavey*

FIGURE 10-4   **Our Data in the General ANOVA Table.**

	No Injury	Minor Injury	Major Injury
Age	5, 25	7, 19, 20, 23, 23	2, 2, 8, 15, 15, 18, 19, 20, 20, 21, 22, 22, 25

FIGURE 10-5   **Statistical Program Output: ANOVA Table.**

ANOVA

Age

	Sum of Squares	df	Mean Square	F	Significance
Between groups	23.908	2	11.954	0.198	0.823
Within groups	1028.892	17	60.523		
Total	1052.800	19			

Where does the *F*-statistic value come from? It is the mean square between groups divided by the mean square within groups or, using data from Figure 10-5:

$$F = \frac{11.954}{60.523} = 0.198$$

Where do the mean squares come from? These are just the sums of squares divided by their respective degrees of freedom. Look at Figure 10-5, and you can see that the following is true:

$$\frac{23.908}{2} = 11.954 \qquad \frac{1028.892}{17} = 60.523$$

(continues)

FROM THE STATISTICIAN *Brendan Heavey*

Now we come to the big question: Where do the sums of squares come from? They are the measurements of the variance components from two different sources:

- How much the cells' means vary around the grand mean
- How much the individual data points vary around their respective cell means

The analysis of variance compares these two measures to derive the F-statistic.

If you want to see ANOVA in action, check out the articles by Chen et al. (2007), Papastavrou et al. (2009), and Zurmehly (2008).

SUMMARY

You are doing a spectacular job at learning these concepts if you made it this far! Let's review the main points from this chapter.

The ANOVA (analysis of variance) is used when comparing the sample means for a single dependent variable among two or more independent groups or samples.

The repeat-measures ANOVA is used to examine a change over time in the same sample population. The test is useful for dependent samples. When using repeat-measures ANOVA, you must be aware of position or latency effects. These effects can occur when a subject is being exposed to more than one treatment over time and the order of the treatments received can impact the outcome in different ways. Also, be aware of carry-over effects, which occur when previous treatments continue to have an effect through the next treatment and the measurement of the dependent variable may not be accurate.

CHAPTER 10 REVIEW QUESTIONS

Questions 1–12: In a study by Vassiliadou et al. (2008), the role of nursing in sexual counseling of myocardial patients was examined. The authors examined professional nurses and collected data about their gender, age, education, unit of employment, and experience in cardiac clinics. They then compared, among other things, the knowledge and comfort level nurses had with regard to sexual counseling. [Reprinted with permission from *The Health Sciences Journal*. Original source is Vassiliadou et al. (2008).]

1. What are the dependent variables?

2. If knowledge is measured by the score in points the nurse receives on a test, is this a quantitative or qualitative variable? Continuous or categorical? What level of measurement is it?

_____

_____

_____

3. These researchers conducted surveys at a nursing conference. What type of sample is this? How does this affect generalizability of the results?

_____

_____

4. Write an appropriate null hypothesis.

_____

_____

5. Write an appropriate alternative hypothesis.

_____

_____

6. The study has an alpha of 0.05 and a power of 80%. The researchers found a relationship between the unit the nurses worked on and the knowledge scores with a p-value of 0.01. What should they conclude?

_____

_____

7. When comparing nurses from different units and their comfort with this type of counseling, they found a p-value of 0.17. What should they conclude about the comfort level of nurses from different units?

_____

_____

8. When comparing nurses from different units and their comfort level with this type of counseling ($p > 0.17$), what is the F-value probably close to?

_____

_____

9. If this conclusion is incorrect, what type of error would the researchers be making?

_____

_____

10. What is the probability of making this type of error?

_____

_____

11. If the researchers think this type of error is occurring, what might they do to fix it?

_____

_____

12. Why is ANOVA an appropriate test for this study?

_____

_____

Questions 13–21: A study by Heyman et al. (2008) examined a sample of 245 elderly individuals living in long-term care facilities. Each had a grade II–IV pressure ulcer. The pressure ulcers were examined at enrollment and then again at 3 and 9 weeks. All of the patients received standard care plus an additional nutritional supplement. The goal of the study was to examine the effects of the nutritional supplement plus routine care on the healing of pressure ulcers in long-term care patients. (See **Figure 10-6**.)

13. What is the dependent variable?

_____

_____

14. What is the independent variable?

_____

_____

_____

15. What level of measurement is the dependent variable?

_____

_____

_____

16. Is it qualitative or quantitative?

_____

_____

17. Is it continuous or categorical?

_____

_____

18. Is the sample independent or dependent?

_____

_____

19. All subjects who met eligibility requirements and consented at 61 long-term care facilities were enrolled with no exclusion criteria. What type of sampling method is this?

_____

_____

20. Write an appropriate null hypothesis.

_____

_____

FIGURE 10-6   **Reduction in Mean Pressure Ulcer Area Achieved With the Oral Nutritional Supplement.**

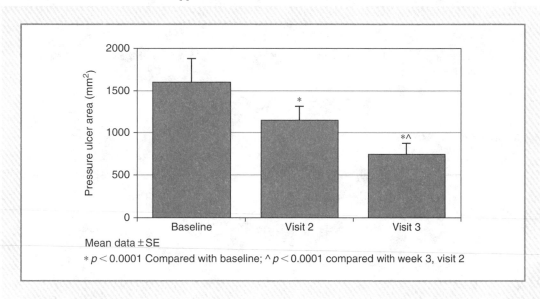

Mean data ± SE

* $p < 0.0001$ Compared with baseline; ^ $p < 0.0001$ compared with week 3, visit 2

21. Write an appropriate alternative hypothesis.

_____

_____

_____

Questions 22–31: Look at Figure 10-6.

22. This study has an alpha of 0.05 and a power of 0.80. Was the size of the pressure ulcer at the first follow-up (visit 2) significantly different from the size at visit 1?

_____

_____

23. Was the size of the pressure ulcer significantly different at the 9-week follow-up (visit 3)?

_____

24. What would you conclude regarding your null hypothesis?

_____

_____

_____

25. What type of error could you be making?

_____

26. What is your chance of making this type of error?

_____

27. As the nurse manager in a long-term care facility, you believe these results are clinically significant. What recommendation would you make in terms of clinical care?

_____

_____

28. Why is repeat-measures ANOVA an appropriate choice for analysis?

_____

_____

29. By using this sample as their own control group, these researchers were able to minimize the effect of differences among the participants and see the effect of the intervention more clearly. This increased what in the study?

_____

_____

30. Using the participants as their own controls minimized the effect of the differences among the participants. How does this affect the sample size needed?

_____

_____

31. Any researcher using repeat-measures ANOVA needs to be aware of position and carry-over effects. What are these? Are they a concern in this study?

_____

FROM THE STATISTICIAN REVIEW QUESTION

32. You are asked to evaluate a nursing program's admission criteria and want to determine whether the mean grade point average (GPA) is different for individuals with higher-ranked letters of recommendation (on a five-point scale: 1 = poor, 5 = excellent). You develop the following ANOVA table:

ANOVA

GPA

	Sum of Squares	df	Mean Square	F	Significance
Between groups	0.686	4			0.316
Within groups	12.122	85			
Total	12.807	89			

Complete the calculations necessary to fill in the rest of the table. What do you conclude?

Questions 33–45: The owners of a large clothing manufacturing plant are considering enacting a footwear policy for employees and have started to gather data on the type of foot coverage worn and injuries. When employees sign in for their shift they now have to indicate the type of foot coverage they are wearing. The occupational health nurse on site believes there is an association between foot injuries and the type of foot coverage worn by the employees in the plant. The nurse decides to evaluate the average number of foot injuries in those wearing open-toed shoes, closed-toed shoes, and steel-toed boots and selects an alpha of 0.05 and a power of 0.80. She is also concerned because the plant has two separate buildings and she wants to make sure her sample is representative of the population and includes equal representation from both buildings.

33. Write appropriate null and alternative hypotheses.

_____

_____

34. What is the dependent variable?

_____

_____

35. What level of measurement is the dependent variable?

_____

_____

36. What test would you use to compare these groups, and why?

_____

_____

37. The nurse divides the population based on the building the employees work in and then randomly selects 50% of the sample from each building for a total of 1,000 subjects in her sample. She then reviews the files of these employees to assess the number of foot injuries and the type of footwear worn at the time of injury in the last 10 days. What type of sample is this? Is it a probability or nonprobability sample?

_____

_____

38. After collecting the data, the nurse creates a bar chart to present the data. What should be on the horizontal and vertical axes in this chart?

_____

_____

39. The nurse finds the following:

Foot Covering	Average Number of Injuries in 10 Days
Open toe	1.47
Closed toe	1.12
Steel toe	0.01

The nurse also wishes to present a grouped frequency table to illustrate the difference in the frequency of injury in steel-toed footwear ($n = 1/211$) vs. non-steel-toed footwear ($n = 42/313$) for the whole population of employees at the plant in the last day of the study ($N = 524$). Show the results.

40. When the nurse analyzes her data she completes an ANOVA comparing the average number of injuries in each of the three groups, and her F-value is $p = 0.001$. What decision should she make about the null? Why?

41. Interpret this result in plain English. Does the nurse know where the statistically significant difference is?

42. The nurse would like to support her argument that all employees should wear steel-toed boots. She now wants to compare the population data for injuries in steel-toed vs. non-steel-toed footwear. What would be an appropriate test to use in this situation? Why?

43. The nurse completes her analysis comparing steel-toed vs. non-steel-toed footwear and injuries. Her p-value is 0.00017. What should she conclude about the null hypothesis? Why?

44. Looking at the grouped frequency data and the significant p-value found in the nurse's t-test to compare the steel-toed vs. non-steel-toed footwear, which group is more likely to experience foot injuries?

45. The nurse presents her results at a national conference where the clinical experts in the field agree these results are critically important to employee health. Are these results clinically significant? Why or why not?

ANSWERS TO CHAPTER 10 REVIEW QUESTIONS

1. Knowledge and comfort level

3. Nonprobability convenience sample; may not be representative; may be a more educated group of nurses or a particularly interested group of nurses

5. Answers may vary; for example, H_1: There is a difference in the knowledge level of nurses working on different units.

7. Fail to reject the null, there is no significant difference.

9. Type two

11. Increase the sample size

13. Pressure ulcer size

15. Collected as ratio-level data, analyzed as ordinal-level data

17. Continuous

19. Nonprobability, convenience sampling

21. Answers may vary; for example, H_1: Pressure ulcers decrease in size by 9 weeks.

23. Yes

25. Type one

27. To give the nutritional supplement

29. Power

31. Position effects (if the order of the interventions affects the outcome) can be avoided by random assignment, and carry-over effects need a wash-out period. Because this study had only one intervention, these are not a concern.

33. Null: There is no relationship between type of foot coverage worn and foot injuries. Alternative null: The average number of foot injuries for those in open-toed, closed-toed, or steel-toed shoes is the same.

35. Ratio

37. Stratified, probability sample

39.

Type of Footwear	Number of Injuries in the Last 48 Hours
Non-steel-toed ($n = 313$)	42
Steel-toed ($n = 211$)	1

41. There is a statistically significant difference among the number of foot injuries in the three groups; however, the nurse cannot determine where the statistically significant difference actually is without further analysis.

43. Reject the null, $p <$ alpha.

45. Yes, it is clinically significant because it is statistically significant and the experts in the field agree it is clinically important as well.

CHAPTER 11

CORRELATION COEFFICIENTS

WHAT ABOUT LOOKING FOR A RELATIONSHIP BETWEEN TWO VARIABLES IN THE SAME SAMPLE?

OBJECTIVES

By the end of this chapter students will be able to:

- Identify situations in which using a correlation coefficient is appropriate.

- Compare correlation coefficients and determine when the requirements of each are met.

- Appropriately match the level of measurement of a variable and the appropriate correlation coefficient test.

- Write null and alternative hypotheses that demonstrate an understanding of the guiding principles of correlation coefficients.

- Evaluate a correlation coefficient, and assess the direction of the relationship.

- Differentiate between the strength and the direction of the relationship.

- Determine whether a correlation is statistically significant.

- Identify and calculate the percentage of variance.

- Explain in plain English what the percentage of variance means, and prepare a public health headline using this information.

- Read and interpret a computer printout with correlation coefficients, identifying whether the correlation coefficient is statistically significant; the direction of the relationship and the strength of the relationship; and stating these results in statistical terms and in plain English.

- Critique a current nursing research article that uses correlation coefficients; interpret the results statistically and in plain English; and prepare a public health report using this information.

KEY TERMS

Chi-square test
The test used to find a relationship or difference in an outcome or a dependent variable measured at the nominal or ordinal level.

Coefficient of determination
The square of Pearson's r (r^2).

Correlation
A relationship between at least two variables.

Direction of the relationship
Either the positive or the negative nature of the relationship. If positive, both variables move in the same direction; if negative, when one variable increases in value the other decreases, and vice versa.

Homoscedasticity
Equal spread of one variable around all the levels of another variable.

Pearson's correlation coefficient (r)
The test used if you are looking for a relationship between two variables that are normally distributed and are at the interval or ratio level.

Percentage of variance
The amount of variance in one variable that is explained by the second variable, determined by multiplying the coefficient of determination by 100.

Spearman correlation coefficient (ρ)
The test used to determine whether there is a relationship between two variables when at least one is ordinal or not normally distributed.

Strength of the relationship
Determined by the absolute value of the correlation coefficient.

LOOKING FOR A RELATIONSHIP IN ONE SAMPLE

Sometimes nurses want to know the relationship or association between two variables in a single sample. For example, is there an association between working overtime hours and medication errors among the nurses in your hospital?

THE NULL AND ALTERNATIVE HYPOTHESES

In this example, you would develop the following null and alternative hypotheses.

H_0: There is no association between overtime hours worked and medication errors.

H_1: There is an association between overtime hours worked and medication errors.

When they did this very study in New York, they found a statistically significant positive relationship between overtime hours worked and medication errors, so they rejected the null hypothesis. The public health laws were changed as a result, and it is now illegal in New York State to mandate a nurse to work overtime beyond a 16-hour shift. Nurses who work shifts longer than this voluntarily (or for the extra income) are held personally responsible for any errors they make due to fatigue or exhaustion (New York State Nurses Association, n.d.). This is an example of looking for a relationship, or **correlation**, between two variables—in this case, hours worked and medication errors.

SELECTING THE BEST CORRELATION TEST TO USE

For the several types of correlation tests, the lead question is the same as it was before: What level of measurement are my variables? Now you can understand why this is such an important question in statistics! The level of measurement of the variables involved in any analysis impacts what you can do with the data and what conclusions you can draw. If, in the relationship you wish to examine, at least one of the variables is only measured at a nominal level, you still need to use the **chi-square test**, but this time you are looking at a relationship between two variables from only one independent sample. (What a flexible test!) However:

- If the lowest level of data collected for at least one variable is measured at the ordinal level or is not normally distributed, you should use the **Spearman correlation coefficient (ρ)** (the Greek letter rho). (You can sometimes use the Pearson's correlation coefficient with ordinal data too, but that is a long story, and you don't need to worry about it now.)
- If you have two variables that are at the interval or ratio data level and they are normally distributed, you can use the **Pearson's correlation coefficient (r)**.

DIRECTION OF THE RELATIONSHIP

Both the Spearman and Pearson's correlation coefficients describe the direction and strength of a linear relationship between two variables. A linear association is represented by a straight line. The **direction of the relationship** is either positive or negative. A positive correlation means that when one variable increases, the other variable does too, and when one decreases, so does the other. Both variables move in the same direction. In a positive correlation, the coefficient (ρ or r) is positive. Let's use every professor's favorite example of a positive relationship. (Yes, we do this for subliminal messaging effect as well.) The relationship between the time spent studying for an exam and the grade received on the exam is usually positively correlated. Conversely, if less time is spent on studying, the grade received is usually lower.

In a negative relationship or correlation, if one variable increases, the second variable decreases and vice versa. For example, the relationship between smoking and life expectancy has a negative correlation. When smoking increases, life expectancy decreases; when smoking decreases, life expectancy increases. In this case, the correlation coefficient (ρ or r) is negative.

SAMPLE SIZE

You must have a sample of at least three subjects for correlation coefficients. If you are looking for a linear relationship between only two measures (subjects) of a variable, you will always find one: You can always connect two points with a straight line (that's why it is called linear). For all of these tests, you need two variables to correlate and at least three subjects in the sample; then you can compute the appropriate correlation coefficient.

STRENGTH OF THE RELATIONSHIP

The **strength of the relationship** or correlation is determined by the absolute value of the correlation coefficient. Absolute value is just the numeric value of a number without the positive or negative indicator. For example, the absolute value of −4 is 4, and the absolute value of +4 is 4.

Correlation coefficients are always between −1 and +1.

- A correlation coefficient of −1 indicates a perfect negative relationship.
- The closer the correlation is to zero, the weaker the relationship is.
- If the correlation is zero, there is no relationship at all. In this case, the variables are completely independent.
- At the other extreme, a correlation coefficient of 1 indicates a perfect positive relationship.
- If the *absolute* value of the correlation coefficient is < 0.3, the relationship between the variables is weak.
- If it is 0.3–0.5, the relationship between the variables is moderate.
- If it is > 0.5, the relationship between the variables is strong.

So, for example, putting the direction and strength concepts together, a correlation coefficient of 0.2 shows a weak positive relationship between the variables. A correlation coefficient of −0.6 shows a strong negative relationship between the variables.

STATISTICAL SIGNIFICANCE

But wait a minute here, do not be fooled. You need to look at something else to determine whether these results are significant. What do you always need to check before you know whether the results are statistically significant? *Yes*—the p-value! Your statistical computing package will give you a corresponding p-value, which determines whether your correlation coefficient is significant. If your sample size is very small, you may have large correlation coefficients that are not significant (*p* > alpha). Even small correlation coefficients can be significant when the sample is large (*p* < alpha).

Nurses usually remember this quite well. I usually remind my class that the last step at the end of a nursing shift (tabulating the patient's intake and output for the shift) and the last step at the end of a statistics test are remarkably similar. You always have to check the "pee" value! You have to know the p-value before you are done with your statistical analysis as well.

APPROPRIATE USE OF CORRELATION COEFFICIENTS

Selecting any test depends on certain assumptions, which for correlation coefficients should include the following:

- First, the sample subjects should be independent and randomly selected.
- Second, the appropriate level of measurement should be met (if at least one variable is nominal, chi-square; if the lowest level of data is ordinal, Spearman's; if both variables are interval/ratio, Pearson's).
- Third, two variables must be compared, and a linear relationship must be present. (You can always check a scatterplot to make sure this is the case.)

- If you wish to use the Pearson's correlation coefficient, both variables should be normally distributed in the population (the fancy term for this is *bivariate normal*) and **homoscedasticity** should be present. Homoscedasticity can be seen visually on a scatterplot. It is a truly horrific word to try to say but its meaning is pretty simple. If the spread of a variable is about the same around all the levels of another variable, this assumption is met. For example, if as each hour of work increases there are 1–2 more nursing errors, homoscedasticity is present. However, if at 5 hours of work 0–3 errors are present, and at 10 hours of work 0–9 errors are reported, and at 15 hours of work 1–15 errors are reported, this assumption is violated. These last two assumptions for the Pearson's correlation coefficient can be violated if the sample size is large enough. The big takeaway message about these assumptions is to make sure your sample has at least 50 subjects. Then you can proceed as long as you have ratio-/interval-level data (Corty, 2007).

Here are some questions to answer before you select the best correlation test:

- Do you have one independent sample?
- Are you looking for a linear relationship between two variables in this sample?
- What is the lowest level of measurement for each of your variables?
  Nominal: Select chi-square.
  Ordinal: Select Spearman's.
  Interval/ratio: Select Pearson's.

When selecting the correlation test, make sure your data meets the test's assumptions.

If it does not, you need to select a test at a lower level. For example, if you wish to use Pearson's correlation coefficient but your sample is only 20 subjects and is not normally distributed, you generally need to use the Spearman's correlation coefficient.

MORE USES FOR PEARSON'S R

You should know one other thing about the Pearson's *r*. If you square it (r^2), it becomes the **coefficient of determination**. If you then multiply it by 100, it tells you something called the **percentage of variance**, which nurses readily understand. The percentage of variance is simply the amount of variance in one variable that is explained by the second variable. For example, suppose you were reading a study that found that daily caloric intake and total serum cholesterol had a statistically significant Pearson's correlation coefficient of 0.7 ($r = 0.7$). You could square this number ($0.7 \times 0.7 = 0.49$) to calculate the coefficient of determination. When you multiply that coefficient by 100, you can then use plain English again: "Forty-nine percent of the differences they found in total serum cholesterol were explained by differences in daily caloric intake."

The other neat piece of information that you can determine with this percentage is the amount of the differences in total serum cholesterol that were related to factors other than daily caloric intake (e.g., genetics, exercise, etc.). That amount is the difference between the percentage of variance and 100%, in this case, $100\% - 49\% = 51\%$. In terms of clinical importance, any value of $r > 0.3$ (which you know means it explains about 9% of the variance) is considered clinically important (Grove, 2007). Now that is pretty understandable!

You can also use the Pearson's correlation coefficient (r) to determine the effect size to use when calculating sample size. Think about it; it makes sense. The effect size is just an estimate of the relationship/difference you are attempting to find.

- When you have a strong correlation, you have a large effect size and don't need such a large sample to find a statistically significant difference if it exists.
- When the strength of the correlation is weak, the effect size is small and you need a larger sample to detect statistically significant differences.

For example, when Pearson's $r = 0.4$, one of your variables explains 16% of the variance in the other, which is considered a medium effect size. When Pearson's $r = 0.6$, one of your variables explains 36% of the variance of the other, which is a large effect size. You will need a larger sample to detect the small or medium correlation (i.e., $r = 0.4$) and a smaller sample when you are trying to detect the large correlation (i.e., $r = 0.6$). (I told you it made sense.)

FROM THE STATISTICIAN   *Brendan Heavey*

Methods: Correlation Coefficients

Here is an example of how to use correlation coefficients. The director of the local community center believes that students are at increased risk for accidental injury as they progress through the higher grades in high school. He wants to know how these two variables (increased risk of accidental injury and grade level) are related in the population that the center serves. He gives you a database with randomly collected surveys of 108 adolescents who participate at the center and asks you to complete an analysis. You note two questions in particular: One asks the student to identify his or her current grade, and another asks how often the student experienced an accidental injury in the last 6 months. Injury risk is coded 1–5: 1 = never, 2 = less than three times, 3 = three to five times, 4 = five to seven times, 5 = more than seven times. You decide to analyze these two variables using a correlation coefficient. Being the statistical genius that you are, you know that identifying the correct correlation coefficient for the job means answering a few questions.

First, do you have one independent sample? In this example, the data you have is all collected from adolescents at one community center. There is no contrasting sample, and you are not dividing the sample into different samples to compare. Each of the adolescents was surveyed only once, and they are not related in any way. Therefore, you have one independent sample.

Second, you need to be sure that you are looking for a linear relationship between two variables, and you are.

Last, you must identify the level of measurement of the variables in order to select the correct correlation coefficient. The first variable is the current grade level of the student, which is interval/ratio level. The level of measurement of injury risk is ordinal (the intervals are not equal so don't be misled by the coding).

(continues)

You can now identify which correlation coefficient is appropriate for this sample. Your statistical program outputs the tables shown in **Figures 11-1** and **11-2**. Which table is appropriate for your analysis, and why?

Because you know your risk variable is ordinal, you know you must use the Spearman ρ correlation coefficient in Figure 11-2. (If it were interval or ratio, you could use the table in Figure 11-1 and the Pearson's correlation coefficient.) Looking at Figure 11-2, you can determine that the correlation between the risk of injury and the student's grade level is actually 0.156. You, of course, also know that the p-value associated with this correlation is 0.106, which is not significant. You are then able to report to the community center director that, unfortunately, the grade level explains only 2.4% (0.156 × 0.156) of the variance in accidental injury in this sample. It is not significantly related to the risk for accidental injury.

Before you wrap this analysis up, go back to Figure 11-2 and make sure you understand what the other numbers mean. Don't worry—they're pretty straightforward. First, you know that $N = 108$ means that 108 adolescents were in your sample. But why is 1.00 listed as the correlation coefficient between grade and grade and between risk and risk? That number shows that, when you correlate a variable with itself, the correlation coefficient is 1.00. It is a perfect correlation. Any variable should correlate perfectly with itself!

FIGURE 11-1	**Correlation Coefficient: Table 1.**

Correlations

		Risk	Grade
Risk	Pearson's correlation	1.000	0.159
	Significance (two-tailed)		0.101
	N	108.000	108
Grade	Pearson correlation	0.159	1.000
	Significance (two-tailed)	0.101	
	N	108	108.000

FIGURE 11-2	**Correlation Coefficient: Table 2.**

			Risk	Grade
Spearman's ρ	Risk	Correlation coefficient	1.000	0.156
		Significance (two-tailed)		0.106
		N	108	108
	Grade	Correlation coefficient	0.156	1.000
		Significance (two-tailed)	0.106	
		N	108	108

SUMMARY

Good job completing the chapter! Now we will review the concepts.

A correlation is the relationship between two variables.

- You use the chi-square test to look for a correlation when you have an independent sample and at least one of the variables you wish to examine is of nominal-level data.
- The Spearman correlation coefficient is used if the variable with the lowest level of data is ordinal or not normally distributed.
- If you have two normally distributed interval- or ratio-level variables, the Pearson's correlation coefficient is used.

Both the Spearman and Pearson's correlation coefficients tell you the direction and strength of the linear relationship between the two variables. The direction of the relationship can be either positive or negative. In a positive correlation, as one variable increases, so does the other; as one variable decreases, so does the other. In a negative correlation, as one variable increases, the second variable decreases; as one variable decreases, the second increases.

The strength of the relationship is determined by the absolute value of the correlation coefficient. The coefficient of determination is represented by r^2 because you must square Pearson's r. The percentage of variance is the amount of variance in one variable that is explained by the second variable, and it is determined by multiplying the coefficient of determination (r^2) by 100.

These concepts may be a little confusing, so review this chapter until you feel completely confident. Keep your head up and continue to study hard. Believe it or not, the concepts eventually sink in as you continue to use them. Do you remember learning how to take a blood pressure? I thought I'd never master the skill, and I felt very, very anxious. Now blood pressures are old hat. Statistics is the same; you just need to practice until the concepts make sense. The more you use them, the clearer they become.

CHAPTER 11 REVIEW QUESTIONS

Questions 1–18: You are asked to conduct a study to determine whether there is an association between consumption of milk proteins and levels of serum antibodies in children with autism. You randomly select 50 children previously enrolled in an autism clinical trial, and they are the sample for the study. You select an alpha of 0.05 and a power of 0.80.

1. Your study measures consumption of milk proteins as a yes-or-no question. It measures serum antibodies as a present-or-not-present question. What level are the two variables?

2. What analysis method do you propose based on this information?

3. Your research partner believes it would be better to measure milk protein consumption as a low/moderate/high question and to quantify the serum antibody level by using the actual amount present. If you take this approach, what analysis method do you propose?

4. The biostatistician in your department recommends you change your milk protein measurement to one that is the number of servings per day. You continue to use the actual quantity of the serum antibodies. You might now recommend what analysis method?

5. Write an appropriate null hypothesis for this study.

6. Write an appropriate alternative hypothesis for this study.

7. Is your sample size large enough to conduct a correlation test? Is it large enough to assume a normal distribution and homoscedasticity?

8. You decide to utilize the measurement variables as recommended by the biostatistician and conduct a Pearson's correlation coefficient test. You determine $r = 0.6$. What must your p-value be for this to be statistically significant?

9. Your p-value is 0.08. Is this significant?

10. What do you conclude?

11. Suppose that you were able to refine your measurement tools and repeat the study. This time you determine you had an r of 0.6 with a p-value of 0.049. What would you conclude?

12. This information would let you know that your original conclusion was actually what type of error?

_____

13. What is the strength of the relationship between consumption of milk proteins and serum antibodies?

_____

14. Is the relationship positive or negative? Interpret this in plain English.

_____

15. In this study, what percentage of variance in serum antibody levels is explained by the consumption of milk proteins in children with autism?

_____

16. How much of the variance is explained by other variables?

_____

17. Is this clinically important?

_____

18. If you were going to use this effect size to determine your sample size for another study, would you expect to need a large or small sample?

_____

Questions 19–24: You develop a screening test to be used for children with autism to detect serum antibodies from milk protein consumption and have the following 2 × 2 table.

	+ Disease	**No Disease**	**Totals**
Positive test	10	2	12
Negative test	3	220	223
Totals	13	222	235

Calculate the following values:

19. Sensitivity:

_____

20. Specificity:

_____

21. Positive predictive value:

_____

22. Negative predictive value:

_____

23. Prevalence:

_____

24. If early treatment helps, is this a good screen?

Questions 25–27: You are asked to complete a study for a small school district that is trying to keep as many students at age-appropriate grade levels as possible. You have a measure of grade level and age for the students, as well as the following statistical programming output from a randomized independent sample.

Correlations

		Age	Grade
Age	Pearson correlation	1.000	0.382*
	Significance (two-tailed)		0.000
	N	108.000	108
Grade	Pearson correlation	0.382*	1.000
	Significance (two-tailed)	0.000	
	N	108	108.000

*Correlation is significant at the 0.01 level (two-tailed).

Correlations

			Age	Grade
Spearman's ρ	Age	Correlation coefficient	1.000	0.378*
		Significance (two-tailed)		0.000
		N	108	108
	Grade	Correlation coefficient	0.378*	1.000
		Significance (two-tailed)	0.000	
		N	108	108

*Correlation is significant at the 0.01 level (two-tailed).

25. What is your sample size?

---

26. What is the appropriate correlation coefficient, and why?

---

27. Are age and grade significantly correlated?

Questions 28–30: A nurse researcher conducts a study to determine if taking a new fertility drug is associated with multiple fetal pregnancies. Her sample includes 500 women who are pregnant in her fertility practice. She selects an alpha of 0.05 and a power of 0.80.

28. If taking the new drug is measured as yes/no, what level of measurement is it?

29. If a multiple fetal pregnancy is also measured as yes/no, what correlation test is appropriate, and why?

30. The researcher reports that $p = 0.044$. What conclusion should the researcher make about the null hypothesis? Why?

Question 31–39: A researcher conducts a study to determine if there is an association between time spent in solitary confinement and depression rates in 120 male prisoners. The alpha is 0.05 and the power is 0.80.

31. If time spent in solitary confinement is measured in total hours, what level of measurement is this variable?

32. If depression is measured on a scale with values from 1 to 10, what level of measurement is the variable?

33. What would be the appropriate correlation test, and why?

34. The study reports that $r = 0.4$. What does this mean in plain English?

35. How much of the variance in depression is explained by hours in solitary confinement?

36. If $p = 0.07$, is the correlation significant? Why or why not?

37. If the hypothesis decision is incorrect, what type of error could it be?

38. If instead the study measured time in solitary confinement as none, infrequent, or regularly, what level of measurement would it be?

39. Would this change the correlation test you would recommend? Why or why not?

ANSWERS TO CHAPTER 11 REVIEW QUESTIONS

1. Both nominal

3. Ordinal/ratio—Spearman's correlation coefficient

5. H_0: There is no association between milk protein consumption and serum antibodies.

7. Yes, it is greater than or equal to 3; yes, it is greater than or equal to 50.

9. No

11. Reject the null; there is a relationship.

13. 0.6 = strong

15. $0.6 \times 0.6 = 0.36 = 36\%$

17. Yes, > 9%

19. $10 \div 13 = 0.77$ or 77%

21. $10 \div 12 = 0.83$ or 83%

23. $13 \div 235 = 0.06$ or 6%

25. 108 students

27. $r = 0.382$, which is significant ($p < 0.01$).

29. Chi-square, both nominal level

31. Ratio

33. Pearson's—both are interval/ratio and sample > 50

35. $r^2 \times 100 = 0.16 \times 100 = 16\%$

37. Type two

39. Yes. The ordinal variable means you would need to do a Spearman's correlation now.

CHAPTER 12

REGRESSION ANALYSIS:

QUANTIFYING AN ASSOCIATION
TO PREDICT FUTURE EVENTS

OBJECTIVES

By the end of this chapter students will be able to:

- Identify the conditions under which regression is an appropriate statistical technique.

- Compare and contrast linear regression, multiple regression, and logistic regression.

- Explain how quantifying an association with a regression equation helps a researcher infer or predict future events.

- Use regression coefficients to interpret how a change in the independent variable affects the predicted value of the dependent variable.

- Contrast positive and negative regression coefficients.

- Discuss when reporting an adjusted R square is more appropriate.

- Interpret the SPSS output utilizing multiple regression; determine whether the model as well as the independent variables are significant; and interpret these results in statistical terms and in plain English.

- Critique an article from current nursing research that utilizes a regression technique; determine whether statistical significance is present; and debate whether clinical recommendations should be made.

KEY TERMS

Adjusted R-squared
Used to avoid overestimating the percentage of variance in the outcome explained by the model, such as when there are a large number of independent variables with a relatively small sample size.

Linear regression
Analyzes the relationship between a single independent variable and a single interval- or ratio-level dependent variable, enabling the researcher to make a prediction about a future outcome based on the research data included in the analysis.

Logistic regression
Analyzes the relationship between multiple independent variables and a single dependent or outcome variable when the outcome is binary (only has two categories).

Multiple regression
A statistical method used to look at the relationship between a dependent variable and multiple independent variables to develop a prediction equation based on the research data included in the analysis.

Odds ratio (OR)
The odds or probability of the outcome occurring divided by the odds or probability of the outcome not occurring.

R-squared change
The change in the percentage of the variance in the outcome variable (R^2) that is explained by the model with the addition of another independent variable.

R-squared value (R^2)
The percentage of the variance in the dependent or outcome variable that is explained by the model.

Regression
A statistical technique that allows the researcher to make a prediction about a future outcome based on the research data included.

Regression coefficient
The b value, which tells you the rate of change in the outcome or dependent variable with a one-unit increase in the corresponding independent variable.

Residual
The amount of prediction error in a regression equation.

Standard error of the estimate
The average amount of error there will be in the predicted outcome using a model.

QUANTIFYING AN ASSOCIATION

It is one thing to recognize statistically significant relationships and another to be able to use that information to begin the process of inferring or predicting future events. In order to do that we first need to quantify the association. Let's look at an example. Most obstetric nurses have read the literature showing a significant relationship between smoking and fetal weight. This is helpful knowledge to have for our pregnant patients. However, if you have a patient who is smoking 10 cigarettes a day and she really doesn't want to quit, she may not think smoking 10 cigarettes a day will have that much of an impact on the size of her baby. Just being able to tell her there is a statistically significant correlation between smoking and fetal weight may not be enough.

You are going to need to use more statistics before you can convince this patient that it is important for her to quit smoking.

You know that correlations measure the strength of associations; now we want to be able to quantify that association, which involves one of my favorite statistical techniques, called **regression**. No, we are not all going to take a moment and relive childhood memories. This is math, remember, but it can still be fun! Regression happens to be a favorite test of mine for one basic reason—developing an accurate regression equation is the first step in being able to predict future events. It is like being a psychic on Halloween—but this time your predictions should actually be true!

Of course, there isn't just one kind of regression analysis so let's start with the most basic, although not one that is used that often in the literature. You need to understand the basics of **linear regression** before you understand the more complex types of regression, so it is a good place to begin.

Linear regression looks for a relationship between a single independent variable and a single interval- or ratio-level dependent variable. (You can sometimes use this technique when you have ordinal-level dependent variables as well, but it gets a little more complicated.) Once the temporality of the relationship is established, you can then make an inference or a prediction about the future value of the dependent variable at a given level of the independent variable. In the fetal weight example, you might use linear regression to see the relationship between the number of cigarettes smoked each day and fetal weight. Maybe knowing, for example, that for every five cigarettes a day she eliminates, her baby will weigh about a half a pound more will help motivate your pregnant patient to decrease her cigarette consumption.

FROM THE STATISTICIAN   *Brendan Heavey*

Statistics, Jerry Springer Style: Now Let's Look at Some Relationships That Aren't Functional!

Regression is a method that allows us to examine the relationship between two or more variables. You may recall another way of exploring the relationship between two variables from earlier in life when you first learned to graph the formula of a line using the formula $Y = mX + b$. Remember what all these letters represent:

Y is the dependent variable, and is displayed on the vertical axis.
X is the independent variable, and is displayed on the horizontal axis.
M is the slope, and represents the amount of change in the Y variable for each unit change in the X variable.
b is the Y-intercept, and it tells us the value of Y when the line crosses the vertical axis ($X = 0$).

(continues)

In this relationship, the value of the variable Y varies according to the value of X based on the values of two constants, or parameters. If you know the values of m, X, and b, you can solve for the value of Y exactly. Let's look at an example. In the graph shown in **Figure 12-1**, you can see three functional relationships between the total cost of three different types of treatment for minor wound infections in June. Treatment 1, outpatient treatment, is cheaper per unit, so there is a more gradual rise in overall cost for each additional treated case. Because all three treatments pass through the origin, their Y-intercepts are all 0. In fact, the only difference between these three lines are their slopes. Their equations are:

Treatment 1 (outpatient)—$250/case: $Y = 250\,X$
Treatment 2 (inpatient medical treatment)—$500/case: $Y = 500\,X$
Treatment 3 (same day surgical treatment)—$750/case: $Y = 750\,X$

This math is all well and good, but things rarely work out this nicely in nature. The problem that usually occurs is the relationship between most variables, just like the relationship between many people, is not functional. Can you guess what term best describes the relationship between almost all variables? Why, *statistical*, of course! You see, the difference between a functional relationship and a statistical relationship is that a statistical relationship accounts for error.

FIGURE 12-1 **Relationship Between Total Cost and Number of Patients Treated (Functional Relationship).**

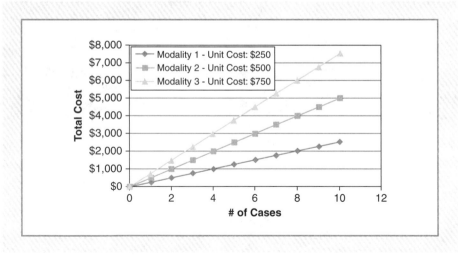

FROM THE STATISTICIAN   *Brendan Heavey*

As it turns out, accounting for error is a very difficult task. We rarely, if ever, know how error is distributed around a mean value, so we usually have to make a few assumptions to allow us to make sense of our data.

In this text, we are doing our best to keep things simple and give you a basic introduction to regression, so we will stick with one of the most basic regression models available, namely the *normal error regression model*. In this model, our most basic assumption is that the error we model is normally distributed around the mean of *Y*. This is okay to do, especially as our sample size is increased. Do you remember why? It is because of the central limit theorem. Because the distribution of the sum of random variables approaches normal as the number of variables is increased, and as our sample size increases, the amount of random error increases, we can assume that the distribution of this random error approaches normality. It is okay to make this assumption as long as you have a large enough sample. It is important to note that a few other assumptions are used in the normal error regression model, but they are beyond the scope of this text and most aspects of life.

So now let's look at what a statistical relationship or *statistical model* looks like. Here is the definition of the normal error regression model:

$$Y_i = \beta_0 + \beta_1 X_i + \varepsilon_i$$

In this model, there are three variables and two parameters (one more than the functional model you just saw). Here is what each of these terms means:

Y_i: The value of the dependent variable in the *i*th observation
X_i: The value of the independent variable in the *i*th observation
ε_i: The normally distributed error variable

β_0 and β_1 are parameters, just like the slope, *m*, and the *Y*-intercept (*b*) were in the functional relationship earlier.

Let's say we now have a little more information on treatment 1 (outpatient management) from our previous example. In this case, although there was an exact functional relationship between number of cases and total cost, when we look at the relationship between unit cost and time, it looks like this:

Cost of Treatment 1 Throughout the Year.

January	$118
February	$150
March	$165
April	$205
May	$215
June	$253

(continues)

FROM THE STATISTICIAN *Brendan Heavey*

Cost of Treatment 1 Throughout the Year.

July	$276
August	$289
September	$310
October	$325
November	$332
December	$362
Avg	$250

There is not an exact functional relationship. In fact, the unit cost is increasing over time but the amount of each increase is different each month. The increase in cost per month varies according to a few different factors, but you can see that if we graph this data, the trendline shows that unit cost is increasing, on average, $21.72 per month (see **Figure 12-2**).

FIGURE 12-2   **Unit Cost by Month for Treatment One.**

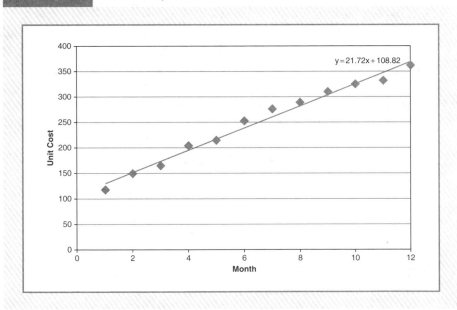

FROM THE STATISTICIAN *Brendan Heavey*

Notice that you can see the error in this relationship. The trendline shows you a functional relationship that is buried inside the statistical relationship. The functional relationship is exactly quantified by two parameters and two variables:

$$Y = 21.72\,X + 108.82$$

The statistical relationship adds a third variable (error, ε), which allows the points on the graph the freedom to vary around this functional relationship, because statistical relationships are never exact:

$$Y = 21.72\,X + 108.82 + \varepsilon$$

Linear regression plots out the values of the dependent variable (i.e., fetal weight) on the y-axis and the values of the independent variable (i.e., daily number of cigarettes) on the x-axis to find the line to best graphically illustrate the relationship between the two variables (see **Figure 12-3**).

Assuming there is a linear relationship (you can see how a trendline is not exactly on the points of data, but the points follow it pretty closely or in a linear fashion), this line can then be used to make predictions about the future value of the dependent variable at the different levels of the independent variable. The difference between where the points of data actually fall and where the line predicts they will fall is something called a **residual**, or the prediction error, which is discussed further in the next From the Statistician. The lower the amount of residual, the better the line fits the actual data points.

The slope of the trendline tells how much the predicted value of the dependent variable changes when there is a one-unit change in the independent variable. In our example, the slope of the line would tell us how much the predicted fetal weight would drop with the consumption of an additional cigarette each day. Seems simple enough, right?

Unfortunately, life is rarely so simple, and statistics has to keep up with it. (And you thought statistics was what made life complicated!) Very rarely is there only one independent variable we need to consider, which may leave you asking: What do you do when you want to predict how two or more variables will affect the dependent or outcome variable? For example, the length of the pregnancy as well as the number of cigarettes smoked each day both affect fetal weight, so you would not want to predict fetal weight with just one of these independent variables, you would want to include both. How can you make an accurate prediction in this situation? (No, no, don't use the crystal ball. . . .) You just need to use another statistical test called **multiple regression**.

FIGURE 12-3 **Fetal Weight at Various Levels of Daily Cigarette Consumption.**

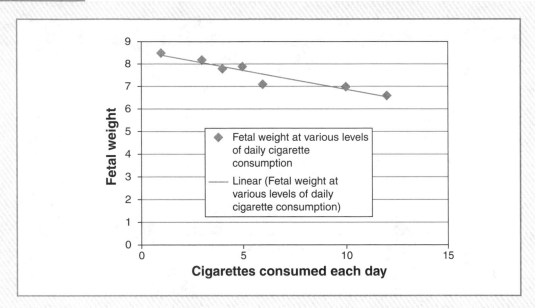

So let's go back to the example of studying fetal weight. Multiple regression lets us take the data we have measuring months pregnant (independent variable #1 or X_1) and the number of cigarettes smoked (independent variable #2 or X_2) and see how these variables relate and affect the outcome, which is fetal weight (dependent variable or Y). Using this example, the relationship can be expressed in an equation like this:

$$Y_i = a + b_1 X_1 + b_2 X_2 + e$$

Now I know many of you just looked at this equation and started to think, what on earth does this equation mean? Don't panic. Let's break it apart.

Y_i is just the value of your dependent variable, in this case how much the fetus weighs.

The value of a is what is called the constant, or the value of Y when the value of X is 0. In our example this would be the value of Y or fetal weight when the patient is not yet 1 month pregnant and has not smoked any cigarettes. Obviously there would still be some fetal weight, although in this example a is probably going to be a very small number.

b_1 is the value of the **regression coefficient** for our first independent variable. It is the rate of change in the outcome for every one-unit increase in the first independent variable. In our example, it is how much we would expect fetal weight to increase for each additional month of pregnancy.

FROM THE STATISTICIAN *Brendan Heavey*

What is a Residual?

Consider the following data, which shows the results of a survey that collected IQ level on a series of patients with elevated blood lead levels.

Obs	BLL (mcg/dL)	IQ
1	7	125
2	18	109
3	22	110
4	25	117
5	29	110
6	37	98
7	44	94
8	56	90
9	64	84
10	100	81

Now, look at what this data looks like when we graph it (see **Figure 12-4**).

Let's look at this model a little more in depth. To do so, we'll need two definitions:

1. We refer to the fitted value of our regression function (or the inferred value of the dependent variable) at a particular X value as $\hat{Y}$ (pronounced Y-hat). Because the formula for our regression line is $Y = -0.4886\,X + 121.4428$, if we are interested in the fitted value at an X of 7, we solve for $\hat{Y}$ like this:

$$\hat{Y} = -0.4886(7) + 121.4428$$
$$= -3.4202 + 121.4428$$
$$= 118.0226$$

This means that at a blood lead level of 7, our regression model infers an IQ of 118.0226 on the y-axis.

2. We refer to the distance between the actual observed value and the regression line as a *residual*, which is usually labeled using the Greek symbol ε. On a graph, it looks like **Figure 12-5**.

(continues)

FROM THE STATISTICIAN *Brendan Heavey*

FIGURE 12-4   **IQ versus BLL.**

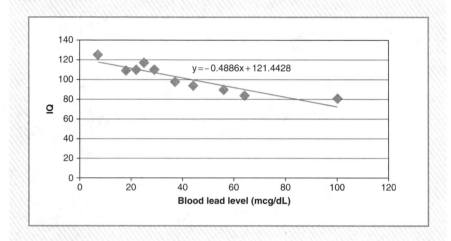

FIGURE 12-5   **Residuals for Figure 12-4.**

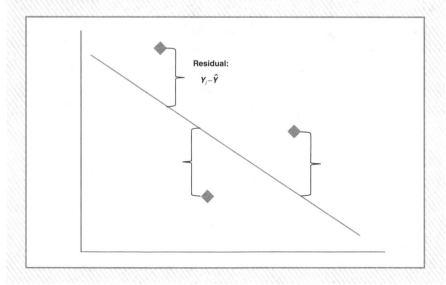

In this example, the fitted regression function equals 118.02 at an X of 7. Now, look at the data we observed to come up with this regression line. The observed value at an X of 7 was 125. Therefore, our residual value at an X of 7 is:

$$\varepsilon = 125 - 118.02 = 6.98$$

Let's look at the data from our example and calculate the residuals for our model. Plug in each of the X's to solve for $\hat{Y}$ and then subtract from the actual observed value to get the residual:

Observation	Blood Lead Level (mcg/dL)	IQ [Y_i]	$\hat{Y}$	Residual
1	7	125	118.02	6.98
2	18	109	112.65	−3.65
3	22	110	110.69	−0.69
4	25	117	109.23	7.77
5	29	110	107.27	2.73
6	37	98	103.36	−5.36
7	44	94	99.94	−5.94
8	56	90	94.08	−4.08
9	64	84	90.17	−6.17
10	100	81	72.58	8.32
			Sum	0

Notice that if you sum the residuals you get a total of 0. This is always true for the normal error linear regression model.

Finally, it is important to point out the distinction between residuals and error. Remember the normal error regression model:

$$Y_i = \beta_0 + \beta_1 X_i + \varepsilon_i$$

It is really easy to confuse the final variable in this model, which represents the error, with residuals. Remember, residuals are a real construct. They are easily calculated from observed data. They represent observed error. The error term in the model is more abstract. It represents all error from the entire model, which has a much larger range than our observed data.

X_1 is the value of our first independent variable, or in this example how many months pregnant the patient is at the time of measurement.

b_2 is the value of the regression coefficient for the second independent variable. It is the rate of change in the outcome for every one-unit increase in the second independent variable. In our example, it is how much change we would expect in fetal weight when one additional cigarette is smoked every day. In all likelihood, the value of b_2 would be negative in this example because increases in daily cigarette consumption usually lower fetal weight. If the value of the regression coefficient is negative, an increase in the corresponding independent variable produces a decrease in the dependent or outcome variable, such as an increase in cigarette consumption producing a decrease in fetal weight.

Last, there is always an error term in statistics, and in this equation it is represented by the e. Just as there are no perfect people, there are no perfect estimates. The e just acknowledges that these statistical procedures are estimates taken from a sample, not the parameters you would find in a population model.

So if we wanted to put the previous equation into plain English using our example, we would say:

Fetal weight = a baseline value + an amount related to the length of the pregnancy + an amount related to the number of cigarettes smoked (probably negative) + a certain amount of error

Now hopefully that makes a little more sense.

Once you put in the data you have about the duration of the pregnancy and the number of cigarettes smoked, assuming this is a good regression equation, you should be able to predict an accurate fetal weight. For example, after we compute the regression equation we determine the following:

$$Y = 0.25 + 0.79\,X_1 - 0.15\,X_2 + 0.5$$

A patient comes into your unit who is having some preterm labor at 7.5 months. She reports smoking 10 cigarettes a day. You might be concerned because you would predict the current fetal weight to be only 5.18 pounds.

$$Y = 0.25 + 0.79(7.5) - 0.15(10) + 0.5$$
$$Y = 5.175 \text{ pounds}$$

Given that information, you might anticipate transferring the patient to a tertiary care facility if you are unable to stop the preterm labor.

Now the next question becomes: How do you know if you have a good regression equation? See, I knew you were going to ask that! Let's look at some computer output to answer that question. There is another piece of good news when it comes to regression analysis, which is that you are not going to do any of the calculations yourself. We are going to make the computer do all the hard work and then we are going to look at the results and see what we have figured out. However, for those of you who like to see the math to help understand the concept, check out the From the Statistician: Methods where you can learn to manually calculate the regression coefficients.

FROM THE STATISTICIAN: METHODS *Brendan Heavey*

Calculating Regression Coefficients (Parameter Estimates)

There are a number of ways to come up with regression coefficients (parameter estimates); the method you probably will choose is to use some computer software package to spit them out. However, I think it is an important exercise to see just what that computer package is doing behind the scenes.

Remember, the normal error simple linear regression model we have been looking at thus far is:

$$Y_i = \beta_0 + \beta_1 X_i + \varepsilon_i$$

This model represents how variables and parameters interact in a population. The true values for the parameters β_1 and β_2 are never really known. However, when we sample real data from a population, we can come up with very good estimates of what these parameters are, given a few reasonable assumptions, by using the following two equations. Notice, we need the result of the first equation to solve the second equation:

$$b_1 = \frac{\sum (X_i - \overline{X})(Y_i - \overline{Y})}{\sum (X_i - \overline{X})^2}$$

$$b_0 = \overline{Y} - b_1 \overline{X}$$

These equations are called the *normal equations* and are derived using a process called *ordinary least squares*.

To calculate these parameters, the first thing we do is find the denominator in the equation for b_1:

$$\sum (X_i - \overline{X})^2$$

This denominator is an example of a very important concept in statistics called a *sum of squares*, which is calculated by subtracting the mean of a set of values from each of the observed values, squaring it, and then summing the results over the whole set. For instance, if we have a dataset with two values:

$$X = \{5, 15\}$$

Our mean value, $\overline{X}, = 10$ and

$$\begin{aligned}
\sum (X_i - \overline{X})^2 &= (5 - 10)^2 + (15 - 10)^2 \\
&= -5^2 + 5^2 \\
&= 25 + 25 \\
&= 50
\end{aligned}$$

(continues)

Notice that a value that is 5 below the mean and a value that is 5 above the mean both get the same amount of weight included in the overall sum (25 each). This sum allows us to quantify the overall distance away from the mean value that our dataset contains, whether that distance is positive or negative.

The concept of a sum of squares is important for a number of reasons, not the least of which is that the equations we use to solve for our regression parameters are derived by calculating all possible sums of squared error in our regression model and selecting the one with the minimum error (also known in calculus as minimizing the sum of squared error). We will revisit the concept of a sum of squares when we learn about multiple regression analysis later in this chapter. Now there is a cliffhanger for you!

For now, let's get back to solving for our estimates of the linear regression model by using data from our last From the Statistician, reproduced here:

Observation	Blood Lead Level (mcg/dL)	IQ [Y_i]
1	7	125
2	18	109
3	22	110
4	25	117
5	29	110
6	37	98
7	44	94
8	56	90
9	64	84
10	100	81

You can see from our formulas that in order to solve for b_1, we need to solve for $\overline{X}$ before we can solve for the sum of squares in the denominator. To do this, simply take the average of all our X's:

$$\overline{X} = \frac{7+18+22+25+29+37+44+56+64+100}{10}$$
$$= \frac{402}{10}$$
$$= 40.2$$

FROM THE STATISTICIAN *Brendan Heavey*

So we now know that in our sample, the average blood lead level (BLL) of the subjects is 40.2 mcg/dL. Now take each individual BLL (X) and subtract the mean BLL ($\overline{X}$) we calculated for the whole sample and square the result (shown here in the third column):

X_i	$X_i - \overline{X}$	$(X_i - \overline{X})^2$
7	−33.2	1102.24
18	−22.2	492.84
22	−18.2	331.24
25	−15.2	231.04
29	−11.2	125.44
37	−3.2	10.24
44	3.8	14.44
56	15.8	249.64
64	23.8	566.44
100	59.8	3576.04

Now, sum the results of $(X_i - \overline{X})^2$:

$$\Sigma(X_i - \overline{X})^2 = 1102.25 + 492.84 + 331.24 + 231.04 + 125.44 + 10.24 + 14.44 + 249.64 + 566.44 + 3576.04$$
$$= 6699.6$$

So, the denominator of our first parameter, b_1, is 6699.6.

Now let's go back and find the numerator of b_1. First solve for the mean value of $Y(\overline{Y})$. To do so, simply add up all the observed IQ values (Y) and divide by the number of observations, 10:

$$\overline{Y} = \frac{125 + 109 + 110 + 117 + 110 + 98 + 94 + 90 + 84 + 81}{10}$$

$$\overline{Y} = 101.8$$

(continues)

FROM THE STATISTICIAN *Brendan Heavey*

Now, subtract $\overline{X}$ from each of the X's and $\overline{Y}$ from each of the Y's:

X_i	$X_i - \overline{X}$	Y_i	$Y_i - \overline{Y}$
7	−33.2	125	23.2
18	−22.2	109	7.2
22	−18.2	110	8.2
25	−15.2	117	15.2
29	−11.2	110	8.2
37	−3.2	98	−3.8
44	3.8	94	−7.8
56	15.8	90	−11.8
64	23.8	84	−17.8
100	59.8	81	−20.8

Now, multiply column 2 by column 4 in the above table and sum the result to get the numerator:

$X_i - \overline{X}$	$Y_i - \overline{Y}$	$(X_i - \overline{X})*(Y_i - \overline{Y})$
−33.2	23.2	−770.24
−22.2	7.2	−159.84
−18.2	8.2	−149.24
−15.2	15.2	−231.04
−11.2	8.2	−91.84
−3.2	−3.8	12.16
3.8	−7.8	−29.64
15.8	−11.8	−186.44
23.8	−17.8	−423.64
59.8	−20.8	−1243.84
$\sum (X_i - \overline{X})(Y_i - \overline{Y})$		−3273.6

FROM THE STATISTICIAN *Brendan Heavey*

Now, take this numerator, −3273.6, and divide by the denominator we solved for before, 6699.6:

$$b_1 = \frac{\sum (X_i - \overline{X})(Y_i - \overline{Y})}{\sum (X_i - \overline{X})^2}$$

$$= \frac{-3273.6}{6699.6}$$

To come up with our first parameter estimate:

$$b_1 = -0.48863$$

Now, because we know b_1, $\overline{Y}$, and $\overline{X}$ we can solve for b_0 pretty easily:

$$b_0 = \overline{Y} - b_0\overline{X}$$

$$= 101.8 - (-0.48862 * 40.2)$$

$$= 101.8 + 19.6429$$

$$= 121.4429$$

And there we have it, our regression equation is:

$$Y_i = 121.4429 - 0.4886 X_i$$

Notice we left out the error term. Do you remember how to calculate the error of the sampled values? The residuals! The residuals represent the distance between our observed values and our calculated regression line. However, because our residuals sum to 0, we can leave that term out when looking at our overall model.

Let's say I am interested in predicting an individual's weight. My study includes information about age and height. When I put that information into the computer and complete a regression analysis, I have the following output.

		Model Summary		
Model	R	R Square	Adjusted R Square	Std. Error of the Estimate
1	0.656[a]	0.430	0.367	31.24864
2	0.922[b]	0.850	0.813	16.99823

[a]Predictors: (Constant), age
[b]Predictors: (Constant), age, height

Let's look at each of these columns and figure out what the information means.

The first row (model 1) is when we only include the independent variable of age in the regression equation. The second row (model 2) is when we include age and then add the second independent variable of height to the model.

R is the multiple correlation coefficient that, when squared, gives you the **R-squared (R^2) value**. Great, you say, and what does that mean? Well, R^2 is important because it tells you the percentage of the variance in the dependent or outcome variable that is explained by the model you have built. In this example, the R^2 of 0.850 on line 2 is when both age (independent variable one) and height (independent variable two) are included in the model. This just means including both age and height explains 85% of the variance seen in weight. See, not so bad. That R^2 is handy!

FROM THE STATISTICIAN *Brendan Heavey*

A Closer Look at *R*-Squared

R-squared is a fantastic tool and is often the single statistic used to determine whether we can use a particular regression model. To derive *R*-squared requires looking at a regression equation from a slightly different view. The output from most statistical packages will show us a table with this view of our model, namely the analysis of variance or ANOVA table. It doesn't matter which package you choose to use, you will get almost all the same information on this table. Here's what the output looks like for the model in our previous example:

	ANOVA[a]				
Model	Sum of Squares	df	Mean Square	F	Sig.
1 Regression	1599.567	1	1599.567	39.985	0.000[b]
Residual	320.033	8	40.004		
Total	1919.600	9			

[a]Dependent Variable: IQ
[b]Predictors: (Constant), BLL

FROM THE STATISTICIAN *Brendan Heavey*

Model	Coefficients[a]				
	Unstandardized Coefficients		Standardized Coefficients		
	B	Std. Error	Beta	t	Sig.
1(Constant)	121.433	3.695	−0.913	32.870	0.000
BLL	−0.489	0.077		−6.323	0.000

[a]Dependent Variable: IQ

The three biggest concepts represented in the top table are:

1. Sum of squares due to regression (SSR)
2. Sum of squares due to error (labeled "Residual" here) (SSE)
3. Total sum of squares

All three represent different reasons why Y values vary around their mean. Check out the diagram shown in **Figure 12-6**, which shows total deviation partitioned into two components, SSR and SSE, for the first observed value:

FIGURE 12-6	**Partitioning the Total Deviation Around $\bar{Y}$.**

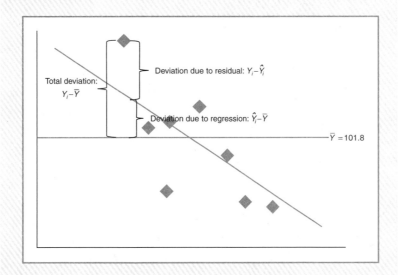

Total deviation: $Y_i - \bar{Y}$

Deviation due to residual: $Y_i - \hat{Y}_i$

Deviation due to regression: $\hat{Y}_i - \bar{Y}$

$\bar{Y} = 101.8$

(continues)

FROM THE STATISTICIAN   *Brendan Heavey*

Here you can see how the total deviation of each observed *Y* value can be partitioned into two parts: the deviation due to the difference between the mean of *Y* and the regression line, and the deviation between the observed value and the regression line. As it turns out, *R*-squared is simply the ratio of the second sum of squares over the total sum of squares.

Some variance is due to the regression itself and some is due to error in the model. Here are the definitions of the sums of squares we're interested in, the total sum of squares (SSTO), the sum of squares due to regression (SSR), and the sum of squares due to error (SSE).

1. $SSTO = \sum (Y_i - \overline{Y})^2$

SSTO represents the sum of the squared distance of each observed *Y* value from the overall mean of *Y*. You can see the distances that are squared and summed in Figure 12-6 under the heading "Total Deviation."

2. $SSR = \sum (\hat{Y}_i - \overline{Y})^2$

SSR represents the sum of the squared distance of the fitted regression line to the overall mean of *Y*. This is the variation that is due to the regression model itself.

3. $SSE = \sum (Y_i - \hat{Y}_i)^2$

SSE represents the sum of the squared distance between the observed *Y* values and the regression line. This is the variation that is due to difference between our observed values and our model, also known as the error in our model.

Let's take a minute and calculate these values by hand for the model in our example.

To calculate SSTO, subtract each observed *Y* from the mean of *Y*, and square that value like this:

SSTO			
IQ [Y_i]	$\overline{Y}$	$Y_i - \overline{Y}$	$(Y_i - \overline{Y})^2$
125	101.8	23.20	538.24
109	101.8	7.20	51.84
110	101.8	8.20	67.24
117	101.8	15.20	231.04
110	101.8	8.20	67.24
98	101.8	−3.80	14.44
94	101.8	−7.80	60.84
90	101.8	−11.80	139.24
84	101.8	−17.80	316.84
81	101.8	−20.80	432.64

FROM THE STATISTICIAN *Brendan Heavey*

Now, sum the right-most column above, and we get our SSTO:

$$SSTO = \sum (Y_i - \overline{Y})^2 = 1919.6$$

To calculate SSR, subtract the mean of Y from the fitted value on our regression line and square it:

SSR			
$\hat{Y}$	$\overline{Y}$	$(\hat{Y} - \overline{Y})$	$(\hat{Y} - \overline{Y})^2$
118.02	101.8	16.22	263.17
112.65	101.8	10.85	117.67
110.69	101.8	8.89	79.09
109.23	101.8	7.43	55.16
107.27	101.8	5.47	29.95
103.36	101.8	1.56	2.44
99.94	101.8	−1.86	3.45
94.08	101.8	−7.72	59.60
90.17	101.8	−11.63	135.24
72.58	101.8	−29.22	853.80

Now, sum the right-most column above and we come up with the SSR:

$$SSR = \sum (\hat{Y} - \overline{Y})^2 = 1599.57$$

To calculate SSE, subtract the value of the regression line from each observed Y value and square it, like this:

SSE			
Y_i	$\hat{Y}$	$(Y_i - \hat{Y}_i)$	$(Y_i - \hat{Y}_i)^2$
125	118.02	6.98	48.69
109	112.65	−3.65	13.30
110	110.69	−0.69	0.48
117	109.23	7.77	60.42

(continues)

FROM THE STATISTICIAN *Brendan Heavey*

SSE			
Y_i	$\hat{Y}$	$(Y_i - \hat{Y}_i)$	$(Y_i - \hat{Y}_i)^2$
110	107.27	2.73	7.44
98	103.36	−5.36	28.77
94	99.94	−5.94	35.32
90	94.08	−4.08	16.64
84	90.17	−6.17	38.08
81	72.58	8.42	70.89

Now, sum the column on the far right to come up with the SSE:

$$SSE = \sum (Y_i - \hat{Y}_i)^2 = 320.03$$

Now we have all the information we need in order to compute R^2. To do so, compute:

$$R^2 = SSR/SSTO = 1599.57 / 1919.6$$
$$= 0.833$$

The section of a printout from SPSS that pertains to R-squared is shown here:

Model Summary				
Model	R	R Square	Adjusted R Square	Std. Error of the Estimate
1	0.913[a]	0.833	0.812	6.32488

[a]Predictors: (Constant), BLL

So, our calculations match . . . hurray!

You will also see the next column, or the **adjusted *R*-squared**, which is sometimes used to avoid overestimating R^2 (the percentage of variance in the outcome explained by the model), particularly when you have a large number of independent variables with a relatively small sample size. In that case, reporting the adjusted *R*-squared would be a better idea. The takeaway idea here is this: If you plan to include a larger number of independent variables you should plan for a larger sample size; otherwise, you are probably overestimating the percentage of variance explained by your regression model (R^2)—and you know the statisticians will not like that!

The **standard error of the estimate** tells you the average amount of error there will be in the predicted outcome (in this case, weight) using this model. (It is the standard deviation of the residuals for those statisticians among you. See From the Statistician: What Is a Residual? to learn more.) In this example, using both age and height as independent variables, the weight

you will predict will be off by an average of approximately 17 pounds. Obviously, you want your prediction to be as accurate as possible, so you would like to see the standard error of the estimate as close to zero as possible.

So now that you know what all of these columns mean, let's go back to the R^2 of 85%, which sounds pretty good. But you know that like all other statistical tests, we still need to look at the *p*-value to see if it is significant. With multiple regression you need to see if the R^2 is significant, but you also need to see if each of the independent variables is significant as well. You could have a significant R^2 with an independent variable that really is not adding anything to the regression model, in which case you wouldn't want to keep that variable in your equation.

Okay, so how do we do all of this? Well, let's take it step by step. If I ask SPSS to tell me the **R-squared change**, I can see what happens to the *R*-squared each time I add another independent variable to the regression model.

| | | | | | Change Statistics | | | | |
| | | | | Model Summary | | | | | |
Model	*R*	*R* Square	Adjusted *R* Square	Std. Error of the Estimate	*R* Square Change	*F* Change	df_1	df_2	Sig. *F* Change
1	0.656[a]	0.430	0.367	31.24864	0.430	6.788	1	9	0.028
2	0.922[b]	0.850	0.813	16.99823	0.420	22.416	1	8	0.001

[a]Predictors: (Constant), age
[b]Predictors: (Constant), age, height

This output shows me that when I added the variable of age, the R-squared went from 0 to 0.43 and it had a p-value of 0.028, which is significant assuming an alpha of 0.05. When I added height to the model (which now includes age and height as independent variables) the R-squared went from 0.43 to 0.85 (from explaining 43% of the variance to explaining 85% of the variance), or a change of 0.42 (42%), which had a p-value of 0.001, which is also significant at an alpha of 0.05. Adding the second independent variable increased the accuracy of predictions made with this model by increasing the amount of variance accounted for by the model.

If we look at the next table SPSS gives us you will see an ANOVA table.

ANOVA[a]					
Model	Sum of Squares	df	Mean Square	F	Sig.
1 Regression	6628.609	1	6628.609	6.788	0.028[b]
Residual	8788.300	9	976.478		
Total	15416.909	10			
2 Regression	13105.391	2	6552.695	22.678	0.001[c]
Residual	2311.518	8	288.940		
Total	15416.909	10			

[a]Dependent Variable: weight
[b]Predictors: (Constant), age
[c]Predictors: (Constant), age, height

In this table you can see the p-value for both the first model (just age included) and the second (age and height included). The first model had a p-value of 0.028 and the second model had a significance level of 0.001.

The last table we see in SPSS shows us the coefficients or the b values in our regression equation.

When we use regression to make predictions, we should look at the column for the unstandardized coefficients (B). First, the B of -584.8 is the constant for our prediction equation. Then you will see the beta coefficients for our independent variables of age and height. This is just the b value in the regression equation. It tells us what a one-unit change in the independent variable will do to the outcome or dependent variable when the other independent variables are held constant. In this example, including both variables in the model gives us $b_1 = 1.712$ and $b_2 = 10.372$. Yikes, we are getting really statistical here—how about a little plain English?

That means when we control for height, every additional year of age adds 1.71 pounds, and when we control for age every additional inch of height adds 10.37 pounds. That should make sense—being taller and getting older both tend to add weight. Not a pretty picture but the reality most of us face anyhow. Both age ($p = 0.010$) and height ($p = 0.001$) are significant, which means even when you control for the other both add to the ability of the model to predict weight. If one of these variables was not significant at this point it would indicate that when we controlled for the other variables, this variable was not significantly adding to the model or did not increase the ability of the model to make an accurate prediction.

Now it is important to note that the order the researcher chooses to enter the variables and interactions between the variables can affect the significance of the variables in question. There are whole books written on these topics so I won't go there in this chapter.

	Coefficients[a]							
	Unstandardized Coefficients		Standardized Coefficients				95.0% Confidence Interval for *B*	
Model	*B*	Std. Error	Beta	*t*	Sig.	Lower Bound	Upper Bound
1 (Constant)	93.552	31.582		2.962	0.016	22.108	164.996
age	2.348	0.901	0.656	2.605	0.028	0.309	4.386
2 (Constant)	−584.801	144.305		−4.053	0.004	−917.568	−252.034
age	1.712	0.508	0.478	3.368	0.010	0.540	2.884
height	10.372	2.191	0.672	4.735	0.001	5.320	15.423

[a]Dependent Variable: weight

Just suffice it to say, researchers shouldn't just enter a bunch of independent variables into the computer and see which ones look significant without a rationale for why they are doing what they are doing.

In our example, the analysis gives us a regression equation we can then use to predict weight.

$$\text{Weight} = -584 + 1.71(\text{years of age})$$
$$+ 10.37(\text{height in inches}) + \text{error}$$

So if a 20-year-old patient was 70 inches tall, you would predict that she might weigh

$$-584 + 1.71(20) + 10.37(70) = 176.1 \text{ pounds}$$

Now I do have to put in one more disclaimer here, which is that making predictions is actually a very complicated process in statistics and what we covered here is really only the first step. For what you need to know at this point, I believe

using the word "prediction" is still the best way to explain the topic, but it probably made a few statisticians twitch. Just remember there is more to come as you go on with your statistics knowledge—such fun to look forward to!

Now there is one last form of regression that I think you should know about and that is **logistic regression**. Remember that multiple regression involves a continuous dependent variable that is at the interval or ratio level. Logistic regression is used when you have a *categorical* dependent variable with two categories (nominal or ordinal with two categories), such as living or dying. (Multinomial logistic regression can be used when the dependent variable has more than two categories, but it is beyond the scope of this text—whew!) One of the advantages of using logistic regression is that the technique generates an **odds ratio (OR)**, which is the odds or probability of the outcome occurring divided by the odds or probability of the outcome not occurring.

FROM THE STATISTICIAN *Brendan Heavey*

Methods: Multiple Regression

To tell you the truth, learning how to estimate parameters in a multiple regression model is not worth the time it would take to learn unless you have a little background in linear algebra. If you happen to have a good sense of working with matrices, I would encourage you to take a full course in regression because most of the fundamentals are exceptionally interesting. In this text, however, we're going to assume that the way you will estimate parameters in regression models with multiple independent variables is by setting up the model in a statistical computing package like SPSS and making the computer perform the calculations for you.

Let's say, for instance, we are interested in expanding our study of the effect blood lead level has on children's IQ. A second variable that we may have some interest in is the IQ of each child's mother. Due to this interest, you might include another question in the study's survey and have data that looks like this:

BLL (mcg/dL)	Mother's IQ	Child's IQ
7	120	125
18	111	109
22	119	110
25	115	117
29	110	110
37	100	98
44	125	94
56	80	90
64	81	84
100	95	81

In this case, we have two independent variables, blood lead level and mother's IQ, and we're interested to see how well we can determine what a child's IQ will be given *both* of these predictors. So, in essence, we want to set up a multiple regression model in SPSS with two independent variables—BLL and mother's IQ—and one dependent variable—child's IQ.

There are two differences in the setup of this model from the one we set up in the last From the Statistician. First, your dataset will have another variable, so it will look like this:

FROM THE STATISTICIAN *Brendan Heavey*

Serum Lead Levels and IQ.

	BII	MothersIQ	IQ
1	7.00	120.00	125.00
2	18.00	111.00	109.00
3	22.00	119.00	110.00
4	25.00	115.00	117.00
5	29.00	110.00	110.00
6	37.00	100.00	98.00
7	44.00	125.00	94.00
8	56.00	80.00	90.00
9	64.00	81.00	84.00
10	100.00	95.00	81.00

Source: Reprint Courtesy of International Business Machines Corporation, © International Business Machines Corporation. SPSS Inc. was acquired by IBM in October, 1999.

Next, when you set up the regression, you will have to add a second variable, MothersIQ, to the list of independent variables, like this:

Adding Independent Variables to a Regression Model using SPSS.

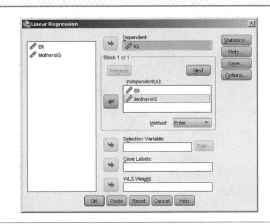

Source: Reprint Courtesy of International Business Machines Corporation, © International Business Machines Corporation. SPSS Inc. was acquired by IBM in October, 1999.

(continues)

The resulting tables will have almost the exact same structure as before with different data. The only really big difference in the structure of the resulting table is that there will now be three parameters in the Coefficients table, which is reproduced here:

			Coefficients[a]			
Model	**Unstandardized Coefficients**		**Standardized Coefficients**		
	B	**Std. Error**	**Beta**	**t**	**Sig.**
1 (Constant)	99.624	21.261		4.686	0.002
BLL	−0.420	0.102	−0.784	−4.132	0.004
Mother's IQ	0.180	0.173	0.198	1.042	0.332

[a]Dependent Variable: IQ

Notice there are three parameters, the *y*-intercept or constant, BLL level, and mother's IQ. Each parameter has a coefficient, which is equivalent to what we would call slope if this were a functional relationship. Therefore, this model can be written as:

$$Y = -0.419556X_1 + 0.180322X_2 + 99.624035 + \varepsilon$$

Note: Please note that by default SPSS shows parameter estimates to three decimal places, but for this example we have performed some magic to get the estimates out to a few more decimals so that the results all tie together.

And you can think of this model as:

$$IQ = -0.419556 \text{ Blood Lead Level} + 0.180322 * \text{Mother's IQ} + 99.624035 + \text{Error}$$

So now, if we're interested in what IQ level this model would result in based on a child with a blood lead level of 7 mcg/dL and a mother's IQ of 120, we would plug these two *X*'s into the regression equation and come up with the following result:

$$\hat{Y}[IQ] = -0.419556 * 7 + 0.180322 * 120 + 99.624035$$
$$\hat{Y} = -2.937 + 21.639 + 99.624$$
$$\hat{Y} = 118.33$$

Based on the same logic, we would come up with the following fitted values for our regression function (in the right-most column):

X_1 BLL (mcg/dL)	X_2 Mother's IQ	IQ [Y_i]	$\hat{Y}$
7	120	125	118.33
18	111	109	112.09
22	119	110	111.85
25	115	117	109.87
29	110	110	107.29
37	100	98	102.13
44	125	94	103.70
56	80	90	90.55
64	81	84	87.38
100	95	81	74.80

Now, something really interesting: Once you calculate all of the $\hat{Y}$'s, the rest of the model equations are exactly the same as in the single predictor case:

$$SSTO = \sum (Y_i - \bar{Y})^2$$

Here are all the numbers we'll need to calculate SSTO:

Y_i	$\bar{Y}$	$(Y_i - \bar{Y})^2$	$(Y_i - \bar{Y})^2$
125	101.8	23.2	538.24
109	101.8	7.2	51.84
110	101.8	8.2	67.24
117	101.8	15.2	231.04
110	101.8	8.2	67.24
98	101.8	−3.8	14.44
94	101.8	−7.8	60.84
90	101.8	−11.8	139.24
84	101.8	−17.8	316.84
81	101.8	−20.8	432.64

(continues)

FROM THE STATISTICIAN *Brendan Heavey*

Now, sum the right-most column:

$$SSTO = 1919.6$$

Next, SSR's formula:

$$SSR = \sum (\hat{Y}_i - \bar{Y})^2$$

And all the data we'll need:

$\hat{Y}_i$	$\bar{Y}$	$(\hat{Y}_i - \bar{Y})$	$(\hat{Y}_i - \bar{Y})^2$
118.33	101.8	16.53	273.11
112.09	101.8	10.29	105.84
111.85	101.8	10.05	101.05
109.87	101.8	8.07	65.16
107.29	101.8	5.49	30.17
102.13	101.8	0.33	0.11
103.70	101.8	1.90	3.63
90.55	101.8	−11.25	126.46
87.38	101.8	−14.42	207.98
74.80	101.8	−27.00	729.05

Sum the right-most column:

$$SSR = 1642.535$$

SSE's formula is:

$$SSE = \sum (Y_i - \hat{Y}_i)^2$$

FROM THE STATISTICIAN *Brendan Heavey*

All the data:

Y_i	$\hat{Y}_i$	$(Y_i - \hat{Y}_i)$	$(Y_i - \hat{Y}_i)^2$
125	118.33	6.67	44.54
109	112.09	−3.09	9.54
110	111.85	−1.85	3.43
117	109.87	7.13	50.80
110	107.29	2.71	7.33
98	102.13	−4.13	17.08
94	103.70	−9.70	94.17
90	90.55	−0.55	0.31
84	87.38	−3.38	11.42
81	74.80	6.20	38.45

Sum the right-most column:

$$SSE = 277.065$$

Which is great, because that's what the output from SPSS tells us in the ANOVA table for this model:

Model	Sum of Squares	df	Mean Square	F	Sig.
ANOVA[a]					
1 Regression	1642.535	2	821.268	20.749	0.001[b]
Residual	277.065	7	39.581		
Total	1919.600	9			

[a]Dependent Variable: IQ
[b]Predictors: (Constant), MothersIQ, BLL

(continues)

FROM THE STATISTICIAN *Brendan Heavey*

Now, let's examine the resulting R^2. We could calculate it ourselves using the same equation as before, substituting the values in the ANOVA table for SSTO and SSR:

$$R^2 = \frac{SSR}{SSTO}$$
$$= \frac{1642.535}{1919.600}$$
$$= 0.856$$

Or, we could just look at the first table produced by SPSS for this model:

Model Summary				
Model	R	R Square	Adjusted R Square	Std. Error of the Estimate
1	0.925[a]	0.856	0.814	6.29132

[a]Predictors: (Constant), MothersIQ, BLL

Finally, let's look back at the R^2 value from the model with one predictor variable:

Model Summary				
Model	R	R Square	Adjusted R Square	Std. Error of the Estimate
1	0.913[a]	0.833	0.812	6.32488

[a]Predictors: (Constant), BLL

Notice, our R^2 went from 0.833 to 0.856 just by adding a second predictor. An R^2 that results from a model with multiple independent variables will always be greater than or equal to the R^2 from any of the models resulting from fewer of these same independent variables. Said a different way, when adding more and more predictors, R^2 will never go down.

SUMMARY

Regression analysis is a statistical procedure that allows us to develop a regression equation that we can use to infer or predict future events. There are several types of regression. In this chapter we discussed linear regression, multiple regression, and logistic regression. Linear regression analyzes the relationship between a single independent variable and a single interval- or ratio-level dependent variable. The slope (b) of the linear regression equation tells us how much the predicted value of the dependent variable changes when there is a one-unit change in the independent variable. The residual is the prediction error or how far away from the prediction line the actual data points fall.

When researchers want to predict how two or more variables affect a dependent variable they may use multiple regression, where the values of the regression coefficients (b) show the change in the dependent variable for a one-unit increase in the independent variable with which it is associated. Each regression model has a corresponding R-squared, which tells you how much of the variance in the dependent variable (outcome) is explained by the independent variables you have included in the model or equation. When sample size is small, researchers sometimes report the adjusted R-squared to avoid overestimating the amount of variance in the dependent variable explained by the independent variables in the equation. The R-squared change tells you the additional variance in the dependent variable accounted for when you add another independent variable. Make sure the R-squared change is statistically significant if you want to increase the accuracy of your prediction equation.

There will always be some error involved in any prediction (yes—even yours!), and with multiple regression we see this estimated by the standard error of the estimate. Researchers try to make the standard error of the estimate as small as possible, obviously trying to make their predictions as accurate as possible.

The last form of regression we discussed was logistic regression, which is used when the outcome or dependent variable is binary, such as for mortality. Logistic regression lets researchers report an odds ratio that tells them the odds or probability of the outcome event occurring in one group versus another.

CHAPTER 12 REVIEW QUESTIONS

Questions 1–4: Mosfeldt et al. (2012) collected data on 792 patients age 60 or over who were admitted to a hospital in Denmark with a hip fracture between 2008 and 2010. They reported that an elevated creatinine level upon hospital admission for a hip fracture (> 90 *mmol*/L for women and >105 *mmol*/L for men) is associated with an almost threefold increase in mortality risk.

1. What is the independent variable? What level of measurement is it?

2. What is the dependent variable? What level of measurement is it?

_____

_____

3. What type of sample is this? Is it a probability or nonprobability sample?

_____

_____

4. These researchers chose to use a regression model. Should they perform a linear regression, multiple regression, or logistic regression? Why?

_____

_____

Questions 5–10: In another study researchers randomly selected five hospitals with orthopedic units in the United States and collected data from all the male patients over age 60 admitted for hip fracture. The researchers then report that admission levels of creatinine and hemoglobin can be used to predict the number of days the patient will need to stay in the hospital.

5. What would be the independent variables? What level are they?

_____

_____

6. What would be the dependent variable? What level is it?

_____

_____

7. What type of sampling method is this? Is it probability or nonprobability sampling?

_____

_____

8. Why might these researchers have chosen to exclude those admitted with a hip fracture who are younger than 60?

_____

_____

9. Would it be appropriate to use these results to predict the length of stay for female patients over age 60 admitted with hip fractures? Why or why not?

_____

_____

10. If these researchers had already established that a causative relationship existed between these variables and asked you for a statistics consultation, what would you tell them is the appropriate regression technique to apply? Explain your answer.

_____

_____

Questions 11–18: Assume that age and academic knowledge (graded exam: 0–100%) have been shown to be related to health knowledge (knowledge questionnaire score: 0–100%) among teens. A nurse researcher would like to use the data she has collected from a random sample of 118 teens living in urban centers of New York to predict their health knowledge. She enters the data she has from their academic knowledge test and their age into SPSS and formulates the following tables from the multiple regression option:

Variables Entered/Removed.[a]

Model[b]	Variables Entered	Variables Removed	Method
1	academic_knowledge, age		Enter

[a]Dependent Variable: health_knowledge
[b]All requested variables entered.

Model Summary

Model	R	R Square	Adjusted R Square	Std. Error of the Estimate	Change Statistics				
					R Square Change	F Change	df_1	df_2	Sig. F Change
1	0.864[a]	0.747	0.743	2.13687	0.747	167.056	2	113	0.000

[a]Predictors: (Constant), academic_knowledge, age

ANOVA[a]

Model	Sum of Squares	df	Mean Square	F	Sig.
1 Regression	1525.629	2	762.814	167.056	0.000[b]
Residual	515.983	113	4.566		
Total	2041.612	115			

[a]Dependent Variable: health_knowledge
[b]Predictors: (Constant), academic_knowledge, age

Coefficients[a]

Model	Unstandardized Coefficients		Standardized Coefficients	t	Sig.
	B	Std. Error	Beta		
1 (Constant)	41.891	3.294		12.716	0.000
age	2.711	0.157	0.853	17.322	0.000
academic_knowledge	−0.023	0.029	−0.039	−0.791	0.430

[a]Dependent Variable: health_knowledge

11. According to the SPSS output, what percentage of the variance in health knowledge is explained by age and academic knowledge?

12. Is the *R*-squared significant? Explain your answer.

13. Should the nurse researcher include both independent variables in her final model? Explain your answer.

14. If the nurse researcher includes both independent variables in her prediction equation, her predicted health knowledge score will be incorrect by an average of how many points?

15. According to this model, every 1-year increase in age results in what change in the health knowledge score?

16. Using this model, if a 15-year-old scored 70 on his academic knowledge exam, what would you expect him to score on his health knowledge exam?

17. What type of sample is this?

18. A researcher working with military officers would like to use the data he has collected from them to predict their health knowledge score based on this research. Would this be an appropriate application of this prediction equation? Why or why not?

Questions 19–21: The nurse researcher in the previous example examined her SPSS output and decided to drop the second independent variable (score on the academic knowledge exam) from her model. Doing so resulted in the following SPSS output.

Variables Entered/Removed[a]

Model	Variables Entered	Variables Removed	Method
1	age[b]	.	Enter

[a]Dependent Variable: health_knowledge
[b]All requested variables entered.

Model Summary

Model	R	R Square	Adjusted R Square	Std. Error of the Estimate
1	0.864[a]	0.746	0.744	2.13337

[a]Predictors: (Constant), age

ANOVA[a]

Model	Sum of Squares	df	Mean Square	F	Sig.
1 Regression	1522.769	1	1522.769	334.582	0.000[b]
Residual	518.844	114	4.551		
Total	2041.612	115			

[a]Dependent Variable: health_knowledge
[b]Predictors: (Constant), age

Coefficients[a]

Model	Unstandardized Coefficients		Standardized Coefficients	t	Sig.
	B	Std. Error	Beta		
1 (Constant)	39.890	2.108		18.920	0.000
age	2.746	0.150	0.864	18.292	0.000

[a]Dependent Variable: health_knowledge

19. Does this model explain more or less of the variance in the health knowledge score? Is this a large change? Does that make sense?

_____

_____

20. In which model is the predicted outcome more accurate?

_____

_____

21. Using this prediction equation, if a 15-year-old scored 70 on his academic knowledge exam, what would you predict he would score on his health knowledge exam?

_____

_____

Questions 22–25: This sample includes 9 teens age 14, 12 teens age 15, 25 teens age 16, 27 teens age 17, and 45 teens age 18.

22. Show this frequency distribution graphically.

_____

_____

23. What level of measurement is age in this example?

_____

_____

24. Calculate all appropriate measures of central tendency for this variable.

_____

_____

25. Is age normally distributed in this sample? Explain your answer.

_____

_____

ANSWERS TO CHAPTER 12 REVIEW QUESTIONS

1. Creatinine level, interval/ratio

3. Convenience, nonprobability

5. Creatinine levels upon admission and hemoglobin levels upon admission, interval/ratio level

7. Cluster sampling, probability sampling

9. No, the sample includes only men so it is not representative of a population of women.

11. R-squared $= 74.7\%$, adjusted R-squared $= 74.3\%$

13. No, beta for age is 2.711 with a significant p-value ($p = 0.000$), whereas the b for academic knowledge is -0.023, which is insignificant ($p = 0.43$).

15. An increase of 2.711 points (unstandardized age coefficient = 2.711)

17. Random or probability sample

19. The model explains slightly less of the variance in the health knowledge score. (R-squared changes from 0.747 to 0.746.) This is not a large change, which makes sense because an independent variable was eliminated in this model but it was an insignificant independent variable so the change should be small.

21. $81.08 = 39.89 + 2.746(15)$

23. Interval

25. No, the mean, median, and mode are not equal; therefore, we know the sample is not normally distributed.

CHAPTER 13

RELATIVE RISK, ODDS RATIO, AND ATTRIBUTABLE RISK

MAKING THE PUBLIC ANNOUNCEMENT

OBJECTIVES

By the end of this chapter students will be able to:

- Define epidemiology.
- Compare and contrast the three major study designs used in epidemiology, and evaluate the strengths and weaknesses of each.
- Compare and contrast incidence data and prevalence data.
- Explain why relative risk is a helpful measure.
- Write null and alternative hypotheses that demonstrate an understanding of relative risk (RR) and the odds ratio (OR).
- Formulate a 2×2 table from a given data set.

- Calculate incidence rates, relative risk, and odds ratios. Interpret relative risks and odds ratios of less than one, equal to one, and greater than one.
- Evaluate whether it is appropriate to calculate a relative risk or an odds ratio from three nursing research proposals.
- Calculate the attributable risk for the exposed group, and interpret it for the exposed group in statistical terms and in plain English.
- Calculate attack rates and determine the likely source of an outbreak.

- Prepare a public health headline that states attributable risk results in language the general population will understand.
- Critique a current nursing research article that utilizes odds ratios, and interpret the results statistically and in plain English.

- Prepare a public health report using odds ratio results in language the general public will understand.
- Interpret SPSS output, and determine whether a given relative risk and odds ratio are significant. Explain these results statistically and in plain English.

KEY TERMS

Attack rate

The incidence rate in the exposed group or the number of cases divided by all those exposed to a particular agent.

Attributable risk for the exposed group (AR$_e$)

The amount of a disease or an outcome in an exposed group that is due to a particular exposure.

Case control study

A study design that starts with the outcome of interest and looks back to determine exposure.

Cohort study

A prospective design that follows a group of individuals over time to see who develops the outcome of interest.

Cross-sectional study

A study design that collects the data about exposure and outcome at the same time.

Epidemiology

The study of the distribution of disease.

Incidence cases

The number of new cases that occur among a sample during the duration of the study.

Odds ratio (OR)

Calculates an approximation of the relative risk using prevalence data (the odds that a case was exposed divided by the odds that a control was exposed).

Prevalence cases

Those cases that already exist in a population.

Protective effect

When an exposure helps prevent a disease (a significant relative risk of less than one).

Relative risk (RR)

The incidence rate in the exposed sample divided by the incidence rate of those not exposed.

Relative risk of one

There is no association between the exposure and the illness.

Risk factor

An exposure that is associated with increased rates of disease.

Risk ratio

Another name for relative risk.

EPIDEMIOLOGY

Nursing is overlapping more and more with **epidemiology**, which is actually the study of the distribution of disease (Gordis, 2000). (Many people, including many who should know better, have no idea what epidemiology is. Although I have a doctorate in epidemiology, on multiple occasions I have been introduced as an endocrinologist!) Epidemiologists like to see how disease is distributed and then ask the age-old question: Why? Some of the tools we use to examine this question in the public health arena are becoming more and more popular in nursing research, so I am going to make sure you are ready to combine what you know as a nurse with what you can learn about epidemiology in this chapter.

STUDY DESIGNS USED IN EPIDEMIOLOGY

There are basically three types of epidemiological studies (and many hybrid versions of them that you don't have to worry about right now):

- Cohort study
- Case control study
- Cross-sectional study

COHORT STUDY

A **cohort study** is a prospective design that follows a group of individuals over time to see who develops the outcome of interest. For example, you might follow the nurses at your hospital to see which, if any, develop osteoporosis. In a cohort study, you start by measuring exposure, and then you monitor

for outcomes. In this study, the exposure you are measuring is consumption of dairy products, and you are monitoring for the outcome of osteoporosis. You also have to eliminate the **prevalence cases**, that is, the nurses who already have the disease you wish to study. Then you conduct an initial survey of the remaining nurses to see what they eat and drink, whether they smoke, whether they lift patients regularly, what unit they work on, how many hours they sleep, and so on. You then monitor the group for 40 years and see who develops osteoporosis, your outcome of interest. You can also look at multiple exposures (diet, smoking, lifting, sleeping, etc.) and determine which, if any, are associated with developing osteoporosis later in life.

One of the advantages of this type of study is that you can monitor for **incidence cases**, which are the new cases that occur among your sample during the duration of your study. That enables you to calculate something called a **relative risk (RR)**, the incidence rate in the exposed sample divided by the incidence rate of those not exposed. The relative risk is also sometimes referred to as the **risk ratio**. So let's try calculating a relative risk. The tricky part is setting up your 2×2 table correctly with the given information. I always suggest having several blank 2×2 tables ready when you have homework or tests coming up, to make sure you have everything ready when you need it.

Suppose there are 1,000 people in a town that was recently devastated by a hurricane. Half the town (500 people) became sick within 2 weeks of the hurricane. It turns out that of the half who got sick, 468 were living in an area where the local water supply was compromised and high bacteria levels were detected. Sixty-three of those who did not get sick lived in this same area with contaminated water. Calculate the RR of becoming sick when "exposed" to living in the area with contaminated water.

In order to determine the RR, you first need to complete a 2 × 2 table and fill in the appropriate cells. Start with the first bit of data you have—the total number of people:

	Disease Present	Disease Absent	Total
Exposed	A	B	
Not Exposed	C	D	
			1000

A = subjects with the exposure and the disease
B = subjects with the exposure and without the disease
C = subjects without the exposure but with the disease
D = subjects without the exposure and without the disease

Then the question tells you that half of the town gets sick, so fill that in:

	Disease Present	Disease Absent	Total
Exposed			
Not Exposed			
	500		1000

This means half of the town does not:

	Disease Present	Disease Absent	Total
Exposed			
Not Exposed			
	500	500	1000

You are then told that of the half that got sick, 468 lived in the exposure area, so fill that in:

	Disease Present	Disease Absent	Total
Exposed	468		
Not Exposed	32		
	500	500	1000

Which means that of those who got sick, 32 were not living in the exposure region because the column must add up to the total number who got sick, or 500.

You are then told that 63 of those who did not get sick lived in the exposure area, so fill that cell in:

	Disease Present	Disease Absent	Total
Exposed	468	63	
Not Exposed	32		
	500	500	1000

Now all that is left to complete your table is a bit of math. The Disease Absent column has to add up to the total at the bottom of 500 (total number who are not sick), so you know there were 437 people who were not living in the exposure area and did not get sick.

	Disease Present	Disease Absent	Total
Exposed	468	63	
Not Exposed	32	437	
	500	500	1000

Then, add up the rows to get your totals in the last columns for those exposed (468 + 63) and those not exposed (32 + 437):

	Disease Present	Disease Absent	Total
Exposed	468	63	531
Not Exposed	32	437	469
	500	500	1000

The last step is to calculate the relative risk, which is the incidence rate in the exposed group divided by the incidence rate in the unexposed group:

$$RR = \frac{\dfrac{A}{A+B}}{\dfrac{C}{C+D}}$$

A = subjects with the exposure and the disease
B = subjects with the exposure and without the disease
C = subjects without the exposure but with the disease
D = subjects without the exposure and without the disease

$$RR = \frac{468/531}{32/437} = \frac{0.88}{0.07} = 12.57$$

In plain English, this means that the group that lived in the area with the contaminated water was 12.57 times as likely to become sick compared to those who lived elsewhere in the town. If the relative risk is greater than one, the group that was exposed has a higher incidence rate than the group that was not. Thus, exposure to the area with the contaminated water may be a risk factor for developing the disease (we still don't know if it is a statistically significant risk factor until we see the p-value or the confidence interval which we will discuss later in the chapter).

Let's look at one more example. In a sample of 300 nurses, you found that, of the 100 nurses who consumed three servings of dairy products daily, only 4 developed osteoporosis. At the same time, among the 200 nurses who did not consume three servings of dairy products daily, 20 developed osteoporosis. We can make a 2 × 2 table to help sort out the results (see **Figure 13-1**).

The incidence cases are all the nurses who developed osteoporosis during the

FIGURE 13-1   **Consumption of Three Dairy Products (Exposure) and Osteoporosis Disease (Disease).**

	Disease	No Disease	Total
Exposed	$A = 4$	$B = 96$	$A + B = 100$
Not exposed*	$C = 20$	$D = 180$	$C + D = 200$
Total	$A + C = 24$	$B + D = 276$	$A + B + C + D = 300$

*Did not consume three dairy products a day.

40-year span of your study: $A + C = 24$. The incidence rate is simply the incidence cases divided by the whole sample times 100: in this case, $24 \div 300 \times 100 = 8\%$. This calculation tells you that 8% of your sample developed osteoporosis during the course of your study. You now need to compare the incidence in the exposed sample to the incidence in the nonexposed sample or the relative risk (RR). The formula is:

$$RR = \frac{\dfrac{A}{A+B}}{\dfrac{C}{C+D}}$$

where

A = subjects with the exposure and the disease
B = subjects with the exposure and without the disease
C = subjects without the exposure but with the disease
D = subjects without the exposure and without the disease

The calculation in this case is:

$$RR = \frac{4/100}{20/200} = \frac{0.4}{0.1}, \text{ or } 40\%$$

The interpretation of this result is that those who were exposed (consumed three servings of dairy a day) were less than half as likely (40% as likely) to develop osteoporosis later in life as those who were not exposed (didn't consume three servings of dairy daily). In this case, the exposure may have had a **protective effect** on disease development.

Interpretations of relative risk include:

- A relative risk of less than one means the group that was exposed had fewer cases develop (lower incidence) than the group that was not exposed. This means the exposure may be a protective factor that helps prevent disease development such as a vaccine.

- A **relative risk of one** indicates that there is no association between the exposure and the illness. For example, you may have found that consuming two cups of fruit juice had no effect on future osteoporosis development; this finding would be reflected by a relative risk of approximately one. The incidence of the disease is the same in the group that was exposed and in the group that was not. There is no relationship between the exposure and the disease.

- If the relative risk is greater than one, the group that was exposed has a higher incidence rate than the group that was not. So the exposure may be a **risk factor** for the development of the disease. For example, suppose in your study you found that the relative risk for smokers was 5.0. This number means that the incidence rate for osteoporosis was five times higher for smokers than for nonsmokers. Put a little differently, those who smoked were five times as likely to develop osteoporosis.

Don't forget that even with a relative risk as high as 5.0, you still need to see whether the number is statistically significant. Statistical significance of the relative risk is once again determined by the *p*-value of the associated chi-square test. You always need to check the *p*. However, sometimes you will see a relative risk reported without the *p*-value stated explicitly. Instead you will see something called confidence intervals or confidence limits.

When you are given the RR that is determined in the study (using a sample) without a *p*-value and a 95% confidence limit is reported, it just means the researcher is 95% sure that the actual RR *in the population* is between these two numbers. (The 95% confidence limits are typically applied and reflect an alpha of 0.05. If there is an alpha of 0.10 you may see 90% confidence limits or intervals reported.) How you interpret the significance of the *p*-value in this situation is not terribly complicated, so let's try it. If in our study there is an RR of 2.3 with a 95% confidence interval of 1.2–3.5, interpreting this value would just mean you are 95% sure that the RR in the population (remember your sample just estimates it) is between 1.2 and 3.5. Anywhere in this range you see a higher rate of disease in the exposed group. Even at the low end, the exposed group is 1.2 times as likely to develop the disease when compared to the unexposed group. This is a situation where the *p*-value is less than alpha and there is a significant relationship between the exposure and the disease; the exposure is a risk factor for the development of the disease anywhere on the continuum of the confidence limits. This means there is a significant difference in the incidence rates between the two groups and is thus a statistically significant RR.

However, if the confidence interval or limits are 0.23–3.59, that would not be the case. Think about what this means and it will make sense. In this case you are 95% certain that the actual RR in the population is between 0.23 and 3.59. If the actual RR is at the bottom end of the confidence interval it would be around 0.23, and the exposed group would have less of the disease than the nonexposed

group (protective exposure). If the RR in the population is 1 (which is included in the 95% confidence interval) then there is no relationship between the exposure and the disease because the disease levels are the same in both the exposed and unexposed groups. If the RR in the population is near the top of the 95% CI then it would be around 3.5, which would mean the exposed group had higher levels of the disease (the exposure is a risk factor). So you are 95% certain that the exposure is either a protective factor, not related, or a risk factor for the disease. How wishy-washy is that? That is how you know you do not have a significant *p*-value. Whenever the confidence limits include the value of one you have an insignificant *p*-value because you are not certain enough to know whether there is a relationship or not. Remember, an RR of one means no relationship, which is your null hypothesis. If the confidence limits include the possibility of the null hypothesis you cannot reject the null hypothesis, which means the *p*-value is greater than your identified alpha and you do not have a statistically significant result.

ATTACK RATES

Now, when you read the newspaper you might notice the journalists referring to epidemics or outbreaks and using the term **attack rate**. Attack rates are used to determine the origin of an outbreak, particularly with foodborne illnesses. You calculate the attack rate by taking all those exposed to the agent of interest and putting that number in the denominator. You then consider, of this group, who got sick and put that number in the numerator. Finally, to make it a percentage you multiply by 100. (That should sound familiar: It is the incidence rate for the exposed group, which is your relative risk numerator. See how these terms relate?)

$$\text{Attack rate} = \frac{\text{Cases in the exposed}}{\text{group (those who got sick)}} \times 100$$
$$\text{All those exposed to that}$$
$$\text{particular agent}$$

Let's look at an example. The health department is investigating an outbreak of salmonella and has determined that many of those with positive stool cultures were at a wedding with 200 people in attendance 2 days earlier. When health department employees interview those at the wedding about what they ate, they determine the information shown in the table.

Exposure of Interest	Number Sick	Number Well	Attack Rate
Caviar	2	45	$\frac{2}{47} \times 100 = 4.3\%$
Alfalfa sprouts	18	24	$\frac{18}{42} \times 100 = 42.9\%$
Humus	1	12	$\frac{1}{13} \times 100 = 7.7\%$
Roast beef	5	43	$\frac{5}{48} \times 100 = 10.4\%$
Chicken	6	32	$\frac{6}{38} \times 100 = 15.8\%$

You can see the attack rates that are associated with the individual food items in the table. The health department investigation team will use this type of table to determine

the probable source of the contamination—which looking at this data, is likely to be the alfalfa sprouts because they have the highest attack rate. The health department will now follow up this piece of information with some additional testing to make a final determination about the cause of the outbreak.

These calculations probably seem very simple, but they can trick you if you are not careful. I always start with the denominator, which may seem a little backwards but that is where most students make their mistake. The denominator of an attack rate is *all* those exposed to the agent, which includes those who are sick and those who are well. When attempting to calculate an attack rate for the caviar, many students will want to start with the number of people who ate the caviar and got sick (which is the correct numerator) but then they put the number of people who ate the caviar and were well in the denominator or they put the whole population in the denominator. (Notice that not everyone at the wedding ate the caviar, so 200 is not the denominator.) I find that starting with the denominator is the best way to avoid this issue. If you begin with who was exposed it helps remind you to include everyone who ate that particular food. You can then go back and figure out, *of that group*, how many subjects got sick.

Let's try another example. At a party there were 203 guests; 27 ate goulash, 36 ate lasagna, and 87 ate shrimp. One hundred and eighty guests consumed alcohol. Seventeen people were sick the next day, including 10 who ate goulash, 7 who ate lasagna, and 30 who ate shrimp.

To use attack rates to determine the likely source of the outbreak, the first thing you need to do is determine the denominator of each attack rate:

- The attack rate for the goulash was 10/27, which means that of the 27 people who ate goulash, 10 were sick. This equals 37%.
- The attack rate for lasagna was 7/36, which means that of the 36 people who ate lasagna, 7 got sick. This equals 19%.
- The attack rate for shrimp was 30/87, which means that of the 87 people who ate shrimp, 30 got sick. This equals 34%.

We cannot determine the attack rate for the alcohol consumption because although we know the denominator (the number at risk) is 180, we don't know how many of them got sick.

We cannot just add up the number who are sick because many of them are in multiple categories. For example, a person who had a shrimp appetizer followed by lasagna and then got sick the next day is counted in both the number who got sick and ate shrimp and the number who got sick and ate lasagna.

Notice that the highest attack rate is associated with the goulash. The item with the highest attack rate is the likely source of the outbreak, so in this situation something in the goulash was the likely source. Notice that although more people who ate shrimp got sick, it is a lower attack rate because a lot of people ate shrimp and didn't get sick. You cannot look at just the absolute numbers; you have to look at percentages.

Sometimes you know the attack rate and need to estimate how many cases are likely to develop in order to allocate resources effectively or plan for necessary prevention and control. For example, if a virus has an attack rate of 10% and there are 45,000 susceptible people in the region, you would anticipate approximately 4,500 cases. Having an idea of how many people are likely to become sick is a very helpful bit of knowledge for public health planning and response.

CASE CONTROL STUDY

A cohort study sounds great, but what about when you can't get a grant to cover the cost of a 40-year prospective trial? Or you are trying to finish a dissertation in less than 40 years? Or if you want to examine a disease that is incredibly rare and may not even show up in a sample of 300 even if you follow them for 40 years? Another study design frequently used in epidemiology, especially when funding is tight or the disease is rare, is called a **case control study**. This type of study starts with the outcome of interest (the disease) and looks back to determine exposure. For example, 10 patients in your hospital have a rapidly progressing case of respiratory failure. All 10 were relatively healthy adults until developing symptoms that included fever and a cough.

You may start your study with this as your sample population (10 cases with similar unusual symptoms) and look back to determine what they may have been exposed to. You interview the patients and their families, review their medical records, and collect data on food consumed, recent travel, occupational exposures, previous illnesses, sexual partners, drug use, and living situations. You also obtain biological specimens. Unfortunately, because you start with those who are already ill (prevalence cases), you cannot calculate an incidence (new cases) rate. However, you can still calculate an approximation of the relative risk, which is the **odds ratio (OR)**: an estimate of the risk of *being* sick, not *becoming* sick (Kahn & Sempos, 1989).

Let's continue with your study of the 10 patients with the unknown disease causing respiratory failure. In addition to your sample of 10 sick patients, you select 10 healthy controls from the community. After completing your interviews and chart reviews, you see that six of the sick patients recently traveled to Eastern Asia and lived in villages where wild birds were raised among the community. Two others worked in a chicken processing plant. Four of your healthy controls also had some type of bird exposure but were not sick. You decide to calculate an OR to see what association may be found between the illness and exposure to some type of bird. You set up another 2 × 2 table (see **Figure 13-2**).

Because this is a case control study, you calculate an OR that divides the odds that a case was exposed by the odds that a control was exposed. Odds and probability are two different things. Odds are the chances that something happens divided by the chance that it doesn't. For example, if the probability of your passing an exam is 80%, the chance that you won't is 20%. The odds of your passing the exam are 80% ÷ 20%, or 4:1 (Gordis, 2000).

To calculate the odds of a case being exposed using a 2 × 2 table, divide A by C. In the example, this would be 8 ÷ 2; in plain English, the odds that a sick patient was exposed to birds are 4:1. The odds of a control being exposed are B ÷ D, or 4 ÷ 6, or 0.66. To get the odds ratio, take 4 ÷ 0.66 to get 6.06. The odds are six times higher that a case (sick patient) was exposed to the birds than a healthy control was. You can do a bit of math and determine that the equation can actually be simplified to

$$\frac{AD}{BC}$$

In this example:

$$\frac{8 \times 6}{4 \times 2} = 6$$

If you find that version easier, you are welcome to do it. If you hate to memorize things (as I do), think about what the OR means and figure out the math from there.

You will see OR and RR used more frequently in the public health and nursing literature because they make for easier understanding by the general public. If you are using the OR to estimate the RR, you can then report that your study *estimates* that individuals exposed to the

FIGURE 13-2   **Exposure to Birds and Respiratory Failure.**

	Cases	Controls	Total
Exposure	A = 8	B = 4	12
No exposure	C = 2	D = 6	8
Total	10	10	20

birds are six times as likely to be sick or that exposure to the birds is associated with an estimated six-fold increase in risk of developing this illness. If these results are significant, they can help the investigator determine the possible causative agent for the respiratory failure by prompting funding for a cohort study or for further investigation. They can also be used to convey public health concerns to the public in a readily understandable way.

You may recall logistic regression, which is the form of regression utilized when the outcome is binary or has only two possibilities, such as alive or dead. One of the reasons researchers like to use logistic regression is that with a little math, the beta values in the prediction equation can be converted to odds ratios. When you see the SPSS output for a logistic regression model you will see a column titled Exp(B). This column indicates the odds ratio associated with that particular exposure and the outcome of interest. Let's consider an example. If a study involving 10,000 subjects reports that having diabetes, having high cholesterol, smoking, and age all affect the probability of being dead upon

arrival at a hospital emergency room, you might see a table such as the one in **Figure 13-3**.

You will see the last column is Exp(B), which is the exponentiation of the beta coefficient otherwise known as the odds ratio for that particular independent variable when all the others are held constant. In other words, having diabetes means a subject is 1.576 times as likely to be dead upon arrival compared to subjects who do not have diabetes when all the other independent variables are held constant or remain the same. In this same example, each yearly increase in age increases the chance of being dead upon arrival 1.03 times. Again, being able to report an OR is helpful when you are trying to explain complicated research to the general public, so someday you, too, may find yourself using logistic regression.

Also, when using the OR to estimate the RR, the results are most accurate when the cases are rare (10% incidence or prevalence), and the cases and controls should be representative of the population in terms of the exposure of interest (Sullivan, 2008). Don't forget the OR is an estimate of the RR, not the same thing; so if you are using

FIGURE 13-3   **Factors Relating to the Chance of Being Dead Upon Arrival in a Hospital Emergency Room ($N = 10,000$).**

Variables in the Equation	B	S.E.	Wald	df	Sig.	Exp(B)
Diabetes	0.455	0.097	21.888	1	0.000	1.576
Cholesterol	0.453	0.059	59.295	1	0.000	1.574
Smoker	0.471	0.065	52.743	1	0.000	1.602
Age	0.030	0.003	88.204	1	0.000	1.031
Constant	−4.124	0.212	377.786	1	0.000	0.016

B = beta coefficient ; S.E. = standard error ; Wald = a type of Chi-square test; df = degrees of freedom ; Sig. = significance of the Wald Chi-Square; Exp(B) = Odds Ratio

this tool incorrectly, your results may not be meaningful.

CROSS-SECTIONAL STUDY

The last type of study frequently used in epidemiology literature is a **cross-sectional study**, which collects the data about exposure and outcome at the same time. For example, suppose you surveyed the nurses on your unit and asked them how many hours they worked that day and if they were tired. You would have data, but not a time sequence. The data is all collected at the same time. This is a significant limiting factor because you cannot determine the direction of the relationship even if you find one. For example, in a survey about work hours and fatigue, you might hypothesize that the hours a nurse works is associated with fatigue; however, with a cross-sectional survey, you cannot assume that the hours worked came before the fatigue. What if the nurse actually came to work fatigued because her spouse is out of work and she deals with a lot of stress at home? She may still work an extra shift that is requested because she needs the additional income, but her fatigue actually started before she came to work. You don't know whether the fatigue is related to the hours worked or to preexisting factors or to factors that contributed to the decision to work extra hours. Cross-sectional studies offer preliminary results and can be useful in forming hypotheses, but they are usually only the beginning of the examination of any significant research issue.

ATTRIBUTABLE RISK

Attributable risk is another concept that makes sense to most nonstatisticians and therefore is a helpful tool when you are disseminating public health information. **Attributable risk for the exposed group (AR_e)** tells you the amount of a disease or outcome in an exposed group that is due to a particular exposure. It is very easy to calculate. The formula is:

AR_e = Incidence rate in the exposed group –
   Incidence rate in the nonexposed group

For example, let's say you develop a cohort study to examine the relationship between tanning bed usage and cataract development. You put your results in the 2 × 2 table shown in **Figure 13-4**. The incidence rate for the

| FIGURE 13-4 | **Tanning Bed Exposure and Cataract Development.** |

	Cataracts	No Cataracts	Totals
Tanning bed usage	60	40	100 (exposed)
No tanning	10	90	100 (nonexposed)
Totals	70 (diseased)	130 (nondiseased)	200

exposed group is 60 per 100. The incidence rate for the unexposed group is 10 per 100. (This is what is considered background risk, or the risk for everyone who does not have the exposure you are looking at.) The attributable risk for the exposed group is the difference: $60/100 - 10/100 = 50/100$, or 50 cases per 100 individuals. If tanning beds were eliminated, you could prevent up to 50 cases of cataracts for 100 individuals who would have tanned before this new policy. (Of course, they could just hit the beaches and lay out in the sun; this is why you can only say *up to* 50 cases.)

To make this number meaningful, determine the proportion of the excess risk (beyond background risk) that is associated with exposure to tanning beds by dividing 50 by 60 (the incidence in the exposed group): 0.83, or 83%. This tells you how much of the risk of cataracts is due to tanning beds in those who used the tanning beds.

How could you use this information clinically? You might advise your patients who tan that, if they stop using the tanning beds, they could reduce their risk of developing cataracts by 83%. That is information that most patients will understand much more easily than if you start talking about incidence and relative risk (Gordis, 2000). It is also the type of information that large populations can understand and that is meaningful to public officials, not to mention making a great headline!

SUMMARY

You have now completed this chapter and should be feeling very confident with this material. To review some key concepts, let's start with epidemiology. Epidemiology is the study of the distribution of disease.

Three types of epidemiological studies are the cohort study, case control study, and cross-sectional study. A cohort study is done by following a group of individuals over time to see who develops the outcome of interest. Remember to exclude prevalence cases in this design because they already have the trait you are studying or wish to study. The incidence data you collect allows you to determine the number of new cases among your sample during the duration of your study.

The relative risk is the incidence rate in the exposed sample divided by the incidence rate of those not exposed. The incidence rate in the exposed sample is the definition of an attack rate. Attack rates are useful in outbreak investigations and can be calculated for many different agents or exposures of interest.

A protective effect occurs anytime you have a significant relative risk less than one. A relative risk of one means that there is no association between the exposure and the illness. An exposure is considered an associated risk factor for the disease when the relative risk is greater than one. Remember for any exposure to be a significant risk or protective factor the *p*-value must be less than alpha or the confidence limits must be entirely above or entirely below 1.

A case control study involves starting with the outcome of interest and working backward to determine exposure. The odds ratio is used to calculate the approximation of the relative risk. You must have incidence data to calculate a relative risk. The odds ratio uses prevalence data (those who are already sick) and estimates relative risk.

In a cross-sectional design, you collect data about exposure and outcomes at the same time.

Public health information has to be delivered in a way that the general public can understand. The results discussed in this chapter may help convert research results into meaningful information for the media and for the general public. People need to be able to understand the important clinical information you have worked so hard to determine!

These new concepts will be helpful to you in mastering statistics, particularly if you are interested in becoming an epidemiologist (a blatant plug for epidemiology).

CHAPTER 13 REVIEW QUESTIONS

Questions 1–9: The variables in **Figure 13-5** have been examined to determine the association with a length of labor.

| FIGURE 13-5 | **Variables Related to Length of Labor > 12 Hours.** |

Variable	RR	95% CI	p-Value
Maternal age < 40			
Yes	0.87	(0.72–1.23)	0.23
No (reference group)	1.00		
Support person present			
Yes	0.43	(0.31–0.56)	0.03
No (reference group)	1.00		
Previous birth			
Yes	0.21	(0.18–0.24)	0.01
No (reference group)	1.00		
Epidural anesthesia			
Yes	1.20	(1.06–1.34)	0.02
No anesthesia or IV/IM anesthesia (reference group)	1.00		

1. What are your "exposure" or independent variables?

_____

_____

2. What is your outcome or dependent variable?

_____

_____

3. If you instead measure your dependent variable rounded to the nearest full hour, what level of measurement is it? Is it quantitative or qualitative?

_____

_____

4. Suppose you originally measured this variable as a yes-or-no response to the question, "Did you feel as though you had a very long labor?" What level of measurement was it? Was it a quantitative or qualitative question?

_____

_____

5. If the study has an alpha of 0.05, which variables are associated with the length of labor? Which are associated with a decreased length of labor? Which are associated with an increased length of labor?

_____

_____

_____

6. Note that when the *p*-value is significant, the RR confidence intervals do not include the value of one. Why?

_____

_____

7. Did maternal age significantly increase the risk of having a labor greater than 12 hours?

_____

_____

8. Did using epidural anesthesia significantly increase the risk of having a longer labor? Compared to whom?

_____

_____

9. Interpret in plain English the RR for maternal age and length of labor.

_____

_____

10. A study reports that children who have breakfast are more likely to pass the fourth-grade math competency (RR = 1.39, 95% CL = 1.30–1.49). You know that because the 95% confidence limits do not include an RR of 1, these results are:

_____

_____

Questions 11–15: A sleep disorder clinic conducted a small cohort study with medical residents working 24-hour shifts to examine how exposure to caffeine, melatonin, strenuous exercise, or television affects the risk of medical residents falling asleep 2 hours later. The results are shown in **Figure 13-6**.

11. What factors are significantly related to the risk of the residents falling asleep?

_____

_____

FIGURE 13-6   **Factors Related to Risk of Falling Asleep 2 Hours After Exposure.**

Variable	RR	95% CI
Caffeine	0.67	0.55–0.75
Melatonin	1.34	1.21–1.46
Exercise	0.88	0.70–1.18
Television	0.93	0.89–0.99

12. What is the dependent or outcome variable?

_____

_____

13. Which exposure had the greatest positive impact on the risk of falling asleep 2 hours after exposure?

_____

14. Interpret the RR for television. Is it significant?

_____

_____

15. Which exposure was most effective in decreasing the risk of falling asleep 2 hours later?

_____

Questions 16–17: The study was replicated, but this time the researchers examined the effect of these exposures on sleep 6 hours later. See **Figure 13-7**.

FIGURE 13-7   **Factors Related to Risk of Falling Asleep 6 Hours After Exposure.**

Variable	RR	95% CI
Caffeine	0.89	0.54–1.51
Melatonin	1.02	0.80–1.45
Exercise	1.34	1.17–2.08
Television	0.96	0.89–0.99

16. Offer a reasonable explanation for the data in the figure.

_____

_____

17. A taxi company wants to implement a policy to diminish the risk of falling asleep behind the wheel. The company has the greatest number of accidents due to drivers falling asleep on the evening shift between 9 and 11 p.m. They are considering either opening the company gym for use by the cab drivers between 1 and 3 p.m. or making free coffee available during the dinner hour (6–7 p.m.). Which policy would this research support implementing?

_____

_____

Questions 18–20: A cohort study following a group of 200 randomly selected adolescent males finds the results shown in **Figure 13-8**.

18. Calculate the incidence rate for traumatic injury.

_____

_____

19. What is the attributable risk for the exposed group? Interpret the risk in plain English.

_____

20. Calculate the RR of traumatic injury for adolescent males who consume alcohol. Assuming your RR is significant, interpret this value.

_____

_____

Questions 21–26: A preschool class visited the zoo. As part of the trip, they had a chance to pet a large lizard and then had lunch. Some students brought lunch from home; others bought lunch at the zoo. That evening four students became ill.

FIGURE 13-8	**Alcohol Use and Traumatic Injury in Adolescent Males.**

	Traumatic Injury	No Traumatic Injury	Totals
Alcohol use	98	40	138
No alcohol use	10	52	62
Totals	108	92	200

Exposure and Disease Status for Preschool Investigation

Student	Pet the Lizard	Lunch	Sick
1	Yes	Home	Yes
2	No	Home	No
3	No	Home	No
4	Yes	Zoo	Yes
5	Yes	Home	Yes
6	No	Zoo	No
7	Yes	Home	No
8	Yes	Zoo	Yes

21. What is the attack rate associated with petting the lizard?

_____

_____

22. What is the attack rate associated with bringing lunch from home?

_____

_____

23. What is the attack rate associated with buying lunch at the zoo?

_____

_____

24. Is petting the lizard, lunch from home, or lunch from the zoo the likely source of the contamination? Explain your answer.

_____

_____

25. If petting the lizard is the source of the contamination, how do you explain student #7?

_____

_____

26. If there were a student who got sick but did not pet the lizard, does this mean petting the lizard is not the source of contamination? What other explanations could there be?

_____

_____

Questions 27–33: You are an infectious disease expert interested in determining if administering tuberculosis (TB) treatment with a directly observed therapy (DOT) program impacts the risk of developing multiple-drug-resistant (MDR) tuberculosis. You randomly select 120 individuals newly diagnosed with TB and randomize them into two equal groups—one group receives treatment without DOT and one group receives treatment with DOT. You follow the groups for 2 years and identify all cases of MDR TB that develop. You find that 2 of the individuals who receive treatment and DOT develop MDR TB, and 10 of the individuals who receive treatment without DOT develop MDR TB.

27. Is this a probability or nonprobability sample?

28. Instead of randomly assigning the groups into those who receive DOT and those who do not, the researcher instead identified a group that received DOT and a group that did not and observed the two groups for a period of 10 years to see who developed MDR TB. What type of epidemiologic or observational study design is this study?

29. Complete the appropriate 2 × 2 table.

30. What is the RR of developing MDR TB?

31. Interpret the RR in plain English.

32. If the 95% CL were 0.12–0.45, is this result significant?

33. Is DOT a risk factor or a protective factor?

ANSWERS TO CHAPTER 13 REVIEW QUESTIONS

1. Maternal age < 40, having a support person present, previous births, and epidural anesthesia

3. Interval, quantitative

5. Having a support person present (decreased risk of labor > 12 hours), having had previous births (decreased risk of labor > 12 hours), and using epidural anesthesia (increased risk of labor > 12 hours)

7. No, RR is not significant.

9. Answers will vary. For example, maternal age less than 40 years is not significantly associated with the risk of labor > 12 hours.

11. Caffeine, melatonin, television

13. Melatonin increased falling asleep 2 hours later.

15. Caffeine

17. Free coffee! Exercise 6 hours before going on shift would increase the number of times the cab drivers fell asleep, whereas coffee 2 hours before the shift would decrease it.

19. $98 \div 138 - 10 \div 62 = 0.71 - 0.16 = 0.55$ or 55%. Fifty-five out of 100 of the cases of injuries in adolescent men are in adolescents who consume alcohol.

21. 4/5 or 80%

23. 2/3 or 66.7%

25. Answers will vary, but may include that the student may have washed his or her hands or his or her immune system may have been strong enough to destroy any contamination ingested.

27. Probability sample

29.

	Disease Positive	No Disease	Row Totals
Exposure to DOT	2	58	60
No Exposure	10	50	60
Column Totals	12	108	120

31. The group who received DOT was less likely (or only 20% as likely) to develop MDR TB compared to those who did not receive DOT. If you would rather put it in terms of not having DOT, those who did not have DOT were 5.57 [RR = (10/60)/(2/60)] times as likely to develop MDR TB compared to those who did receive DOT.

33. A protective exposure

APPENDIX A

TABLES FOR REFERENCE

TABLE 1	*t* Table. Table entries are values of *t* random variables.										
Cumulative probability	0.75	0.80	0.85	0.90	0.95	0.975	0.99	0.995	0.9975	0.999	0.9995
Upper-tail probability	0.25	0.20	0.15	0.10	0.05	0.025	0.01	0.005	0.0025	0.001	0.0005
1	1.000	1.376	1.963	3.078	6.314	12.71	31.82	63.66	127.3	318.3	636.6
2	0.816	1.061	1.386	1.886	2.920	4.303	6.965	9.925	14.09	22.33	31.60
3	0.765	0.978	1.250	1.638	2.353	3.182	4.541	5.841	7.453	10.21	12.92
4	0.741	0.941	1.190	1.533	2.132	2.776	3.747	4.604	5.598	7.173	8.610
5	0.727	0.920	1.156	1.476	2.015	2.571	3.365	4.032	4.773	5.893	6.869
6	0.718	0.906	1.134	1.440	1.943	2.447	3.143	3.707	4.317	5.208	5.959
7	0.711	0.896	1.119	1.415	1.895	2.365	2.998	3.499	4.029	4.785	5.408
8	0.706	0.889	1.108	1.397	1.860	2.306	2.896	3.355	3.833	4.501	5.041
9	0.703	0.883	1.100	1.383	1.833	2.262	2.821	3.250	3.690	4.297	4.781
10	0.700	0.879	1.093	1.372	1.812	2.228	2.764	3.169	3.581	4.144	4.587
11	0.697	0.876	1.088	1.363	1.796	2.201	2.718	3.106	3.497	4.025	4.437
12	0.695	0.873	1.083	1.356	1.782	2.179	2.681	3.055	3.428	3.930	4.318
13	0.694	0.870	1.079	1.350	1.771	2.160	2.650	3.012	3.372	3.852	4.221
14	0.692	0.868	1.076	1.345	1.761	2.145	2.624	2.977	3.326	3.787	4.140
15	0.691	0.866	1.074	1.341	1.753	2.131	2.602	2.947	3.286	3.733	4.073
16	0.690	0.865	1.071	1.337	1.746	2.120	2.583	2.921	3.252	3.686	4.015
17	0.689	0.863	1.069	1.333	1.740	2.110	2.567	2.898	3.222	3.646	3.965
18	0.688	0.862	1.067	1.330	1.734	2.101	2.552	2.878	3.197	3.610	3.922

degrees of freedom

(continues)

TABLE 1							*t* Table. Table entries are values of *t* random variables. *(continued)*				
Cumulative probability	**0.75**	**0.80**	**0.85**	**0.90**	**0.95**	**0.975**	**0.99**	**0.995**	**0.9975**	**0.999**	**0.9995**
Upper-tail probability	**0.25**	**0.20**	**0.15**	**0.10**	**0.05**	**0.025**	**0.01**	**0.005**	**0.0025**	**0.001**	**0.0005**
19	0.688	0.861	1.066	1.328	1.729	2.093	2.539	2.861	3.174	3.579	3.883
20	0.687	0.860	1.064	1.325	1.725	2.086	2.528	2.845	3.153	3.552	3.850
21	0.686	0.859	1.063	1.323	1.721	2.080	2.518	2.831	3.135	3.527	3.819
22	0.686	0.858	1.061	1.321	1.717	2.074	2.508	2.819	3.119	3.505	3.792
23	0.685	0.858	1.060	1.319	1.714	2.069	2.500	2.807	3.104	3.485	3.768
24	0.685	0.857	1.059	1.318	1.711	2.064	2.492	2.797	3.091	3.467	3.745
25	0.684	0.856	1.058	1.316	1.708	2.060	2.485	2.787	3.078	3.450	3.725
26	0.684	0.856	1.058	1.315	1.706	2.056	2.479	2.779	3.067	3.435	3.707
27	0.684	0.855	1.057	1.314	1.703	2.052	2.473	2.771	3.057	3.421	3.690
28	0.683	0.855	1.056	1.313	1.701	2.048	2.467	2.763	3.047	3.408	3.674
29	0.683	0.854	1.055	1.311	1.699	2.045	2.462	2.756	3.038	3.396	3.659
30	0.683	0.854	1.055	1.310	1.697	2.042	2.457	2.750	3.030	3.385	3.646
40	0.681	0.851	1.050	1.303	1.684	2.021	2.423	2.704	2.971	3.307	3.551
60	0.679	0.848	1.045	1.296	1.671	2.000	2.390	2.660	2.915	3.232	3.460
80	0.678	0.846	1.043	1.292	1.664	1.990	2.374	2.639	2.887	3.195	3.416
100	0.677	0.845	1.042	1.290	1.660	1.984	2.364	2.626	2.871	3.174	3.390
1000	0.675	0.842	1.037	1.282	1.646	1.962	2.330	2.581	2.813	3.098	3.300
z	0.674	0.842	1.036	1.282	1.645	1.960	2.326	2.576	2.807	3.090	3.291
Confidence level	**50%**	**60%**	**70%**	**80%**	**90%**	**95%**	**98%**	**99%**	**99.5%**	**99.8%**	**99.9%**

degrees of freedom

t values computed with Microsoft Excel 9.0 TINV function.

TABLE 2

F table. Table entries are *F* values with right-tail probability *P*.

df_2	P	\multicolumn{11}{c}{Degrees of freedom in numerator (df_1)}										
		1	2	3	4	5	6	7	8	12	24	1000
1	0.100	39.86	49.50	53.59	55.83	57.24	58.20	58.91	59.44	60.71	62.00	63.30
	0.050	161.4	199.5	215.7	224.6	230.2	234.0	236.8	238.9	243.9	249.1	254.2
	0.025	647.8	799.5	864.2	899.6	921.8	937.1	948.2	956.7	976.7	997.2	1017.7
	0.010	4052	4999	5403	5625	5764	5859	5928	5981	6106	6235	6363
	0.001	405284	499999	540379	562500	576405	585937	592873	598144	610668	623497	6363011
2	0.100	8.53	9.00	9.16	9.24	9.29	9.33	9.35	9.37	9.41	9.45	9.49
	0.050	18.51	19.00	19.16	19.25	19.30	19.33	19.35	19.37	19.41	19.45	19.49
	0.025	38.51	39.00	39.17	39.25	39.30	39.33	39.36	39.37	39.41	39.46	39.50
	0.010	98.50	99.00	99.17	99.25	99.30	99.33	99.36	99.37	99.42	99.46	99.50
	0.001	998.50	999.00	999.17	999.25	999.30	999.33	999.36	999.37	999.42	999.46	999.50
3	0.100	5.54	5.46	5.39	5.34	5.31	5.28	5.27	5.25	5.22	5.18	5.13
	0.050	10.13	9.55	9.28	9.12	9.01	8.94	8.89	8.85	8.74	8.64	8.53
	0.025	17.44	16.04	15.44	15.10	14.88	14.73	14.62	14.54	14.34	14.12	13.91
	0.010	34.12	30.82	29.46	28.71	28.24	27.91	27.67	27.49	27.05	26.60	26.14
	0.001	167.03	148.50	141.11	137.10	134.58	132.85	131.58	130.62	128.32	125.93	123.53
4	0.100	4.54	4.32	4.19	4.11	4.05	4.01	3.98	3.95	3.90	3.83	3.76
	0.050	7.71	6.94	6.59	6.39	6.26	6.16	6.09	6.04	5.91	5.77	5.63
	0.025	12.22	10.65	9.98	9.60	9.36	9.20	9.07	8.98	8.75	8.51	8.26
	0.010	21.20	18.00	16.69	15.98	15.52	15.21	14.98	14.80	14.37	13.93	13.47
	0.001	74.14	61.25	56.18	53.44	51.71	50.53	49.66	49.00	47.41	45.77	44.09
5	0.100	4.06	3.78	3.62	3.52	3.45	3.40	3.37	3.34	3.27	3.19	3.11
	0.050	6.61	5.79	5.41	5.19	5.05	4.95	4.88	4.82	4.68	4.53	4.37

(continues)

Degrees of freedom in denominator (df_2)

TABLE 2

F table. Table entries are F values with right-tail probability P. (continued)

df_2	P	Degrees of freedom in numerator (df_1)										
		1	2	3	4	5	6	7	8	12	24	1000
	0.025	10.01	8.43	7.76	7.39	7.15	6.98	6.85	6.76	6.52	6.28	6.02
	0.010	16.26	13.27	12.06	11.39	10.97	10.67	10.46	10.29	9.89	9.47	9.03
	0.001	47.18	37.12	33.20	31.09	29.75	28.83	28.16	27.65	26.42	25.13	23.82
6	0.100	3.78	3.46	3.29	3.18	3.11	3.05	3.01	2.98	2.90	2.82	2.72
	0.050	5.99	5.14	4.76	4.53	4.39	4.28	4.21	4.15	4.00	3.84	3.67
	0.025	8.81	7.26	6.60	6.23	5.99	5.82	5.70	5.60	5.37	5.12	4.86
	0.010	13.75	10.92	9.78	9.15	8.75	8.47	8.26	8.10	7.72	7.31	6.89
	0.001	35.51	27.00	23.70	21.92	20.80	20.03	19.46	19.03	17.99	16.90	15.77
7	0.100	3.59	3.26	3.07	2.96	2.88	2.83	2.78	2.75	2.67	2.58	2.47
	0.050	5.59	4.74	4.35	4.12	3.97	3.87	3.79	3.73	3.57	3.41	3.23
	0.025	8.07	6.54	5.89	5.52	5.29	5.12	4.99	4.90	4.67	4.41	4.15
	0.010	12.25	9.55	8.45	7.85	7.46	7.19	6.99	6.84	6.47	6.07	5.66
	0.001	29.25	21.69	18.77	17.20	16.21	15.52	15.02	14.63	13.71	12.73	11.72
8	0.100	3.46	3.11	2.92	2.81	2.73	2.67	2.62	2.59	2.50	2.40	2.30
	0.050	5.32	4.46	4.07	3.84	3.69	3.58	3.50	3.44	3.28	3.12	2.93
	0.025	7.57	6.06	5.42	5.05	4.82	4.65	4.53	4.43	4.20	3.95	3.68
	0.010	11.26	8.65	7.59	7.01	6.63	6.37	6.18	6.03	5.67	5.28	4.87
	0.001	25.41	18.49	15.83	14.39	13.48	12.86	12.40	12.05	11.19	10.30	9.36
9	0.100	3.36	3.01	2.81	2.69	2.61	2.55	2.51	2.47	2.38	2.28	2.16
	0.050	5.12	4.26	3.86	3.63	3.48	3.37	3.29	3.23	3.07	2.90	2.71
	0.025	7.21	5.71	5.08	4.72	4.48	4.32	4.20	4.10	3.87	3.61	3.34
	0.010	10.56	8.02	6.99	6.42	6.06	5.80	5.61	5.47	5.11	4.73	4.32
	0.001	22.86	16.39	13.90	12.56	11.71	11.13	10.70	10.37	9.57	8.72	7.84

Degrees of freedom in denominator (df_2)

Degrees of freedom in numerator (df_1)

df_2	α											
10	0.100	3.29	2.92	2.73	2.61	2.52	2.46	2.41	2.38	2.28	2.18	2.06
	0.050	4.96	4.10	3.71	3.48	3.33	3.22	3.14	3.07	2.91	2.74	2.54
	0.025	6.94	5.46	4.83	4.47	4.24	4.07	3.95	3.85	3.62	3.37	3.09
	0.010	10.04	7.56	6.55	5.99	5.64	5.39	5.20	5.06	4.71	4.33	3.92
	0.001	21.04	14.91	12.55	11.28	10.48	9.93	9.52	9.20	8.45	7.64	6.78
12	0.100	3.18	2.81	2.61	2.48	2.39	2.33	2.28	2.24	2.15	2.04	1.91
	0.050	4.75	3.89	3.49	3.26	3.11	3.00	2.91	2.85	2.69	2.51	2.30
	0.025	6.55	5.10	4.47	4.12	3.89	3.73	3.61	3.51	3.28	3.02	2.73
	0.010	9.33	6.93	5.95	5.41	5.06	4.82	4.64	4.50	4.16	3.78	3.37
	0.001	18.64	12.97	10.80	9.63	8.89	8.38	8.00	7.71	7.00	6.25	5.44
14	0.100	3.10	2.73	2.52	2.39	2.31	2.24	2.19	2.15	2.05	1.94	1.80
	0.050	4.60	3.74	3.34	3.11	2.96	2.85	2.76	2.70	2.53	2.35	2.14
	0.025	6.30	4.86	4.24	3.89	3.66	3.50	3.38	3.29	3.05	2.79	2.50
	0.010	8.86	6.51	5.56	5.04	4.69	4.46	4.28	4.14	3.80	3.43	3.02
	0.001	17.14	11.78	9.73	8.62	7.92	7.44	7.08	6.80	6.13	5.41	4.62
16	0.100	3.05	2.67	2.46	2.33	2.24	2.18	2.13	2.09	1.99	1.87	1.72
	0.050	4.49	3.63	3.24	3.01	2.85	2.74	2.66	2.59	2.42	2.24	2.02
	0.025	6.12	4.69	4.08	3.73	3.50	3.34	3.22	3.12	2.89	2.63	2.32
	0.010	8.53	6.23	5.29	4.77	4.44	4.20	4.03	3.89	3.55	3.18	2.76
	0.001	16.12	10.97	9.01	7.94	7.27	6.80	6.46	6.19	5.55	4.85	4.08
18	0.100	3.01	2.62	2.42	2.29	2.20	2.13	2.08	2.04	1.93	1.81	1.66
	0.050	4.41	3.55	3.16	2.93	2.77	2.66	2.58	2.51	2.34	2.15	1.92
	0.025	5.98	4.56	3.95	3.61	3.38	3.22	3.10	3.01	2.77	2.50	2.20
	0.010	8.29	6.01	5.09	4.58	4.25	4.01	3.84	3.71	3.37	3.00	2.58
	0.001	15.38	10.39	8.49	7.46	6.81	6.35	6.02	5.76	5.13	4.45	3.69

Degrees of freedom in denominator (df_2)

(continues)

TABLE 2 **F table. Table entries are *F* values with right-tail probability *P*. *(continued)***

df₂	P	\multicolumn{11}{c}{Degrees of freedom in numerator (df_1)}

df_2	P	1	2	3	4	5	6	7	8	12	24	1000
20	0.100	2.97	2.59	2.38	2.25	2.16	2.09	2.04	2.00	1.89	1.77	1.61
	0.050	4.35	3.49	3.10	2.87	2.71	2.60	2.51	2.45	2.28	2.08	1.85
	0.025	5.87	4.46	3.86	3.51	3.29	3.13	3.01	2.91	2.68	2.41	2.09
	0.010	8.10	5.85	4.94	4.43	4.10	3.87	3.70	3.56	3.23	2.86	2.43
	0.001	14.82	9.95	8.10	7.10	6.46	6.02	5.69	5.44	4.82	4.15	3.40
30	0.100	2.88	2.49	2.28	2.14	2.05	1.98	1.93	1.88	1.77	1.64	1.46
	0.050	4.17	3.32	2.92	2.69	2.53	2.42	2.33	2.27	2.09	1.89	1.63
	0.025	5.57	4.18	3.59	3.25	3.03	2.87	2.75	2.65	2.41	2.14	1.80
	0.010	7.56	5.39	4.51	4.02	3.70	3.47	3.30	3.17	2.84	2.47	2.02
	0.001	13.29	8.77	7.05	6.12	5.53	5.12	4.82	4.58	4.00	3.36	2.61
50	0.100	2.81	2.41	2.20	2.06	1.97	1.90	1.84	1.80	1.68	1.54	1.33
	0.050	4.03	3.18	2.79	2.56	2.40	2.29	2.20	2.13	1.95	1.74	1.45
	0.025	5.34	3.97	3.39	3.05	2.83	2.67	2.55	2.46	2.22	1.93	1.56
	0.010	7.17	5.06	4.20	3.72	3.41	3.19	3.02	2.89	2.56	2.18	1.70
	0.001	12.22	7.96	6.34	5.46	4.90	4.51	4.22	4.00	3.44	2.82	2.05
100	0.100	2.76	2.36	2.14	2.00	1.91	1.83	1.78	1.73	1.61	1.46	1.22
	0.050	3.94	3.09	2.70	2.46	2.31	2.19	2.10	2.03	1.85	1.63	1.30
	0.025	5.18	3.83	3.25	2.92	2.70	2.54	2.42	2.32	2.08	1.78	1.36
	0.010	6.90	4.82	3.98	3.51	3.21	2.99	2.82	2.69	2.37	1.98	1.45
	0.001	11.50	7.41	5.86	5.02	4.48	4.11	3.83	3.61	3.07	2.46	1.64

Degrees of freedom in denominator (df_2)

Degrees of freedom in numerator (df_1)

1000											
0.100	2.71	2.31	2.09	1.95	1.85	1.78	1.72	1.68	1.55	1.39	1.08
0.050	3.85	3.00	2.61	2.38	2.22	2.11	2.02	1.95	1.76	1.53	1.11
0.025	5.04	3.70	3.13	2.80	2.58	2.42	2.30	2.20	1.96	1.65	1.13
0.010	6.66	4.63	3.80	3.34	3.04	2.82	2.66	2.53	2.20	1.81	1.16
0.001	10.89	6.96	5.46	4.65	4.14	3.78	3.51	3.30	2.77	2.16	1.22

Note: ^{F} values computed with Microsoft Excel 9.0 FINV function.

TABLE 3	**Chi-square table.**

| | Probability in right tail ||||||||||
df	0.975	0.25	0.20	0.15	0.10	0.05	0.025	0.01	0.005	0.001	0.0005
1	0.00098	1.32	1.64	2.07	2.71	3.84	5.02	6.63	7.88	10.83	12.12
2	0.051	2.77	3.22	3.79	4.61	5.99	7.38	9.21	10.60	13.82	15.20
3	0.216	4.11	4.64	5.32	6.25	7.81	9.35	11.34	12.84	16.27	17.73
4	0.48	5.39	5.99	6.74	7.78	9.49	11.14	13.28	14.86	18.47	20.00
5	0.83	6.63	7.29	8.12	9.24	11.07	12.83	15.09	16.75	20.52	22.11
6	1.24	7.84	8.56	9.45	10.64	12.59	14.45	16.81	18.55	22.46	24.10
7	1.69	9.04	9.80	10.75	12.02	14.07	16.01	18.48	20.28	24.32	26.02
8	2.18	10.22	11.03	12.03	13.36	15.51	17.53	20.09	21.95	26.12	27.87
9	2.70	11.39	12.24	13.29	14.68	16.92	19.02	21.67	23.59	27.88	29.67
10	3.25	12.55	13.44	14.53	15.99	18.31	20.48	23.21	25.19	29.59	31.42
11	3.82	13.70	14.63	15.77	17.28	19.68	21.92	24.72	26.76	31.26	33.14
12	4.40	14.85	15.81	16.99	18.55	21.03	23.34	26.22	28.30	32.91	34.82
13	5.01	15.98	16.98	18.20	19.81	22.36	24.74	27.69	29.82	34.53	36.48
14	5.63	17.12	18.15	19.41	21.06	23.68	26.12	29.14	31.32	36.12	38.11
15	6.26	18.25	19.31	20.60	22.31	25.00	27.49	30.58	32.80	37.70	39.72
16	6.91	19.37	20.47	21.79	23.54	26.30	28.85	32.00	34.27	39.25	41.31
17	7.56	20.49	21.61	22.98	24.77	27.59	30.19	33.41	35.72	40.79	42.88
18	8.23	21.60	22.76	24.16	25.99	28.87	31.53	34.81	37.16	42.31	44.43
19	8.91	22.72	23.90	25.33	27.20	30.14	32.85	36.19	38.58	43.82	45.97
20	9.59	23.83	25.04	26.50	28.41	31.41	34.17	37.57	40.00	45.31	47.50
21	10.28	24.93	26.17	27.66	29.62	32.67	35.48	38.93	41.40	46.80	49.01
22	10.98	26.04	27.30	28.82	30.81	33.92	36.78	40.29	42.80	48.27	50.51
23	11.69	27.14	28.43	29.98	32.01	35.17	38.08	41.64	44.18	49.73	52.00
24	12.40	28.24	29.55	31.13	33.20	36.42	39.36	42.98	45.56	51.18	53.48
25	13.12	29.34	30.68	32.28	34.38	37.65	40.65	44.31	46.93	52.62	54.95
26	13.84	30.43	31.79	33.43	35.56	38.89	41.92	45.64	48.29	54.05	56.41
27	14.57	31.53	32.91	34.57	36.74	40.11	43.19	46.96	49.64	55.48	57.86
28	15.31	32.62	34.03	35.71	37.92	41.34	44.46	48.28	50.99	56.89	59.30
29	16.05	33.71	35.14	36.85	39.09	42.56	45.72	49.59	52.34	58.30	60.7

TABLE 3	**Chi-square table.**

	Probability in right tail										
df	**0.975**	**0.25**	**0.20**	**0.15**	**0.10**	**0.05**	**0.025**	**0.01**	**0.005**	**0.001**	**0.0005**
30	16.79	34.80	36.25	37.99	40.26	43.8	47.0	50.9	53.7	59.7	62.2
40	24.43	45.62	47.27	49.24	51.81	55.76	59.34	63.69	66.77	73.40	76.09
50	32.36	56.33	58.16	60.35	63.17	67.50	71.42	76.15	79.49	86.66	89.56
60	40.48	66.98	68.97	71.34	74.40	79.08	83.30	88.38	91.95	99.61	102.69
80	57.15	88.13	90.41	93.11	96.58	101.88	106.63	112.33	116.32	124.84	128.26
100	74.22	109.1	111.7	114.7	118.5	124.3	129.6	135.8	140.2	149.4	153.2

Note: Chi-square values computed with Microsoft Excel 9.0 CHINV function.

REFERENCES

Agresti, A. (2002). *Categorical data analysis* (2nd ed.). Wiley Series in Probability and Statistics. Hoboken, NJ: Wiley.

Anifantaki, S., Prinianakis, G., Vitsaksaki, E., Katsouli, V., Mari, S., Symianakis, A., et al. (2009). Daily interruption of sedative infusions in an adult medical-surgical intensive care unit: Randomized controlled trial. *Journal of Advanced Nursing, 65*(5), 1054–1060.

Chen, M., Shiao, Y., & Gau, Y. (2007). Comparison of adolescent health-related behavior in different family structures. *Journal of Nursing Research, 15*(1), 1–10.

Chung, Y. C., & Hwang, H. L. (2008). Education for homecare patients with leukemia following a cycle of chemotherapy: An exploratory pilot study [online exclusive]. *Oncology Nursing Forum, 35*(5), E86–E87.

Cohen, J. (1988). *Statistical power analysis for the behavioral sciences* (2nd ed.). Hillsdale, NJ: Lawrence Erlbaum.

Corless, I., Lindgren, T., Holzemer, W., Robinson, L., Moezzi, S., Kirksey, K., et al. (2009). Marijuana effectiveness as an HIV self-care strategy. *Clinical Nursing Research, 18*(2), 172–193.

Corty, E. W. (2007). *Using and interpreting statistics: A practical text for the health, behavioral and social sciences*. St. Louis: Mosby.

Doering, L., Cross, R., Magsarili, M., Howitt, L., & Cowan, M. (2007). Utility of observer-rated and self-report instruments for detecting major depression in women after cardiac surgery. *American Journal of Critical Care, 16*(3), 260–269.

Fallovollita, J., Luisi, A. J., Jr., Michalek, S. M., Valverde, A. M., deKemp, R. A., Haka, M. S., et al. (2006). Prediction of arrhythmic events with positron emission tomography. *Contemporary Clinical Trials, 27*(4), 374–388.

Fowler, J., Jarvis, P., & Chevannes, M. (2002). *Practical statistics for nursing and health care.* Chichester, UK: John Wiley & Sons.

Gordis, L. (2000). *Epidemiology* (2nd ed.). Philadelphia: W. B. Saunders.

Grove, S. K. (2007). *Statistics for health care research: A practical workbook.* St. Louis: W. B. Saunders.

Heyman, H., Van De Looversosch, D., Jeijer, E., & Schols, J. (2008). Benefits of an oral nutritional supplement on pressure ulcer healing in long-term care. *Journal of Wound Care, 17*(11), 476–480.

Johnson, N. L., & Kotz, S. (1997). *Leading personalities in statistical sciences.* Wiley Series in Probability and Statistics. Hoboken, NJ: Wiley.

Kahn, H., & Sempos, C. (1989). *Statistical methods in epidemiology.* New York: Oxford University Press.

Munro, B. H. (2005). *Statistical methods for health care research* (5th ed.). Philadelphia: Lippincott Williams & Wilkins.

New York State Nurses Association. (n.d.). Mandatory overtime law. Retrieved from http://www.nysna.org/practice/mot/intro.htm.

Nieswiadomy, R. (2008). *Foundations of nursing research* (5th ed.). Upper Saddle River, NJ: Pearson Education.

Norman, G. R., & Streiner, D. L. (2008). *Biostatistics: The bare essentials* (3rd ed.). Hamilton, ON, Canada: BC Decker.

Oepkes, D., Seaward, P. G., Vandenbussche, F. P., Windrim, R., Kingdom, J., Bevene, J., et al. (2006). Doppler ultrasonography versus amniocentesis to predict fetal anemia. *New England Journal of Medicine, 355*(2), 156–164.

Olbrys, K. M. (2001). The effect of topical lidocaine anesthetic on reported pain in women who undergo needle wire localization prior to breast biopsy. *Southern Online Journal of Nursing Research, 6*(2), 1–18.

Pagano, M., & Gauvreau, K. (1993). *Principles of biostatistics.* Belmont, CA: Wadsworth.

Papastavrou, E., Tsangari, H., Kalokerinou, A., Papacostas, S., & Sourtzi, P. (2009). Gender issues in caring for demented relatives. *Health Science Journal, 3*(1), 41–53.

Plichta, S. B., & Garzon, L. S. (2009). *Statistics for nursing and allied health.* Philadelphia: Wolters Kluwer Health/Lippincott Williams & Wilkins.

Schilling, F., Spix, C., Berthold, F., Erttmann, R., Fehse, N., Hero, B., et al. (2002). Neuroblastoma screening at one year of age. *New England Journal of Medicine, 346*(14), 1047–1053.

Sullivan, L. M. (2008). *Essentials of biostatistics in public health.* Sudbury, MA: Jones & Bartlett.

Szklo, M., & Nieto, F. J. (2000). *Epidemiology: Beyond the basics.* Gaithersburg, MD: Aspen.

Tobian, A., Serwadda, D., Quinn, T. C., Kigozi, G., Gravitt, P. E., Laeyendecker, O., et al. (2009). Male circumcision for the prevention of HSV2 and HPV infection and syphilis. *New England Journal of Medicine, 360*(13), 1298–1309.

U.S. Department of Labor, Bureau of Labor Statistics. Registered nurses. *Occupational Outlook Handbook*. Retrieved from http://www.bls.gov/ooh/healthcare/registered-nurses.htm.

Vassiliadou, A., Stamatopoulou, E., Triantafyllou, G., Gerodimou, E., Toulia, G., & Pistolas, D. (2008). The role of nurses in the sexual counseling of patients after myocardial infarction. *Health Science Journal, 2*(2), 111–118.

Watson, R., Atkinson, I., & Egerton, P. (2006). *Successful statistics for nursing and healthcare*. Basingstoke, UK: Palgrave Macmillan.

Zellner, K., Boerst, C., & Tabb, W. (2007). Statistics used in current nursing research. *Journal of Nursing Education, 46*(2), 55–59.

EPILOGUE

You've completed the book—I know there is a collective sigh of relief happening right now! I hope you are more comfortable and confident in your ability to understand statistics. You've successfully covered a lot of material and have mastered a great deal of math and statistical concepts. Even if you started this course with some trepidation, I hope you now see you are quite capable of and have been doing math quite well throughout this course. I hope you also realize that statistics can be helpful to your practice as a nurse and that you have the potential to contribute to the growing need for evidence-based practice in our profession. I hope this book helped make the process as painless as possible, and that someday you, too, may become a nurse who "crunches numbers" to help care for your patients in the best way possible. Thank you for allowing me to join you on this journey. I wish you all the best as you go forth in your professional nursing career.

Beth

INDEX